Health and Wellbeing of India's Young People

Shalini Bharat • Geeta Sethi
Editors

Health and Wellbeing of India's Young People

Challenges and Prospects

Springer

Editors
Shalini Bharat
Director, Tata Institute of Social Sciences
Mumbai, Maharashtra, India

Geeta Sethi
Centre of Excellence on Adolescents and Youth
Tata Institute of Social Sciences
Mumbai, Maharashtra, India

ISBN 978-981-13-6592-8 ISBN 978-981-13-6593-5 (eBook)
https://doi.org/10.1007/978-981-13-6593-5

This Springer imprint is published by the registered company Springer Nature Singapore Pte Ltd.
The registered company address is: 152 Beach Road, #21-01/04 Gateway East, Singapore 189721, Singapore

Acknowledgments

A volume of this nature would not have been possible without the valuable contributions of the authors of individual chapters. We acknowledge their hard work and commitment to undertaking rigorous reviews of various thematic streams along with a critical examination of policies and programs for India's adolescents and youth.

We appreciate the contribution of Sahana Mitra to the background research for an overview of the situation of adolescents and youth in India.

Alpana Thadani deserves special appreciation for ably supporting us in the preparation of this volume.

Finally, we acknowledge the contribution of the United Nations Population Fund for their support to the Tata Institute of Social Sciences-UNFPA Centre of Excellence on Adolescents and Youth. The reviews that form the basis for the chapters of this volume were undertaken as part of the work of the center.

Shalini Bharat
Geeta Sethi

Contents

About the Editors and Contributors

Editors

Shalini Bharat is Director of the Tata Institute of Social Sciences, Mumbai, India. She teaches in the Centre for Health and Social Sciences, School of Health Systems Studies of the Institute.

Geeta Sethi served as Senior Coordinator, Centre of Excellence on Adolescents and Youth, Tata Institute of Social Sciences, Mumbai, India. She has earlier served the UN system in various capacities.

Contributors

Lamia Bagasrawala Tata Institute of Social Sciences, Mumbai, India

Swati Banerjee Centre for Livelihoods and Social Innovation, School of Social Work, TISS, Mumbai, India

Chetna Duggal School of Human Ecology, Tata Institute of Social Sciences, Mumbai, India

Saurabh Rai School of Health Systems Studies, Tata Institute of Social Sciences, Mumbai, India

Sunil D. Santha Centre for Livelihoods and Social Innovation, School of Social Work, TISS, Mumbai, India

Devisha Sasidevan Centre for Livelihoods and Social Innovation, School of Social Work, TISS, Mumbai, India

Deepa Shokeen Centre for Excellence on Adolescents & Youth, Tata Institute of Social Sciences, Mumbai, India

Hemal Shroff Centre for Excellence on Adolescents & Youth, Tata Institute of Social Sciences, Mumbai, India

M. Sivakami Center for Health and Social Sciences, School of Health Systems Studies, Tata Institute of Social Sciences, Mumbai, India

Abbreviations

AFHC	Adolescent Friendly Health Clinics
AHD	Adolescent Health Day
ANM	Auxiliary Nurse Midwife
DMHP	District Mental Health Programme
ICMR	Indian Council of Medical Research
LSE	Life Skills Education
MDG	Millennium Development Goals
MoHFW	Ministry of Health and Family Welfare
MO	Medical Officer
NIMHANS	National Institute of Mental Health and Neurosciences
NMHP	National Mental Health Programme
NRHM	National Rural Health Mission
PE	Peer Education
RKSK	Rashtriya Kishor Swasthya Karyakram
SDG	Sustainable Development Goals
TISS	Tata Institute of Social Sciences
UNFPA	United Nations Population Fund
NIMHANS	National Institute of Mental Health and Neurosciences
NSSO	National Sample Survey Office

List of Figures

List of Tables

List of Boxes

Chapter 1
Adolescents and Youth: Setting the Context

Geeta Sethi and Shalini Bharat

Abstract Adolescence and youth are increasingly recognised as significant stages in development that have not received the attention required. The definitions of these phases are not precise, and early childhood and old age have been a priority as health was more precarious at these times of the life cycle. This chapter provides an overview of adolescence and youth and seeks to make a case for why additional attention to this subpopulation is necessary. This takes into consideration demographic and developmental factors as well as those related to health and well-being. The chapter then considers the overall situation of adolescents and youth, with emphasis on the gaps or lags in information as well as in progress. The importance of informed and strategic investment in young people is explored. Finally, this introductory chapter provides a brief outline of the structure of the rest of the book.

Keywords Adolescents · Youth · Demographic · Health · Heterogeneity · Information gaps · Investing

1.1 Introduction

Adolescence is a period of developmental transition that constitutes the movement from childhood to adulthood and which is characterised by remarkable physical, psychological and social changes. The biological maturation that marks this phase of life is accompanied by the consolidation of psychological, sexual and emotional identity and a sense of personhood and 'self'. When individuals enter adolescence, they are largely dependent on nurturing adults for their food, shelter, safety and security and major decisions concerning residence, association, finance and day-to-day activities. By the time they cross the threshold into adulthood, they are in the

G. Sethi (✉)
Centre of Excellence on Adolescents and Youth, Tata Institute of Social Sciences, Mumbai, Maharashtra, India
e-mail: geeta.sethi@tiss.edu

S. Bharat
Director, Tata Institute of Social Sciences, Mumbai, Maharashtra, India

S. Bharat, G. Sethi (eds.), *Health and Wellbeing of India's Young People*,
https://doi.org/10.1007/978-981-13-6593-5_1

prime of their life, at the peak of physical strength, performing productive roles and often providing support to older persons and younger children. This remarkable transition is essential for the continuity and healthy development of communities and countries, whereby productive functions as well as responsibility for governance, cultural heritage and social capital can be seamlessly passed on to the next generation and adapted to changing contexts, ideologies and technologies. In the recent times, with a progressive fall in the age of puberty as well as longer periods of education and training and a delay in marriage and starting families, the period of adolescence and youth has become longer, and its importance for sustained progress is increasingly recognised as a cornerstone for effective national planning and sustainable development programmes.

1.2 Adolescence: The Phase of Growth and Transition

The term 'adolescence' was first used in the fifteenth century and is derived from the Latin word 'adolescere' which meant 'to grow into maturity or to grow up' (Lerner 1993). It is defined as the period of psychosexual development between puberty and adulthood (Erikson 1959) when young people extend their relationships beyond parents and family and are intensely influenced by their peers and the outside world (Jain 2014; Sivagurunathan et al. 2015; Sunitha and Gururaj 2014). At this stage of development, broad demographic, institutional and technological forces play a strong formative role (Saraswathi and Dutta 1988). The chronological period covered by adolescence, even though imprecise, is usually considered to include those between 10 and 19 years of age (Way 2014). This age range, according to Stang and Story (2005), can be further divided into early adolescence (10–14 years), middle adolescence (15–17 years) and late adolescence (18–21 years). In practice, there is still a lack of consensus on the age span that covers the phase of adolescence, and different ages are sometime clubbed with childhood and sometimes with adulthood. This lack of clarity on the age span might be a reflection of inadequate knowledge about the special developmental needs during childhood and adolescence and how they merge with the general privileges of adulthood (Saraswathi and Oke 2013).

Adolescence is marked by change and consolidation. Adolescents go through powerful hormonal changes which can affect emotions and moods strongly. As a result, they can be extremely sensitive, especially to peer opinions and parental censure. Their need to belong and their sense of inadequacy, shame and stigma are very high, and psychological hurt at this age can have a lasting impact on their personality. The adolescent period not only brings changes to bodies but also creates new vulnerabilities to health, both physical and mental, and to human rights abuses, particularly in the arenas of sexuality, marriage and child-bearing (UNFPA 2015). One of the major achievements of adolescence is the development of a sense of identity, of self, based on internalised values, norms and cultural constructs that then guide perceptions and decisions through life (Apter 2013). This makes it crucial that young people are provided with maximum understanding and care (Jain 2014). With the widespread use of social media, the number and diversity of peers with whom adolescents regularly interact has grown exponentially. Not only does this determine the range and content of material that adolescents are exposed to but also affects parental oversight and guidance in terms of their ability to supervise the use of social media.

Overtime, a consensus has emerged among academicians, both social (Arnett 2000; Chaudhary and Sharma 2012; Saraswathi 1999; Schlegel and Barry 1991; Verma and Saraswathi 2002) and biological/medical (Johnson et al. 2009) and across different cultural settings including India, regarding the significance of adolescence as a distinct stage in life that needs to be investigated and understood with seriousness and rigour.

1.3 Youth: The Phase of Intimacy and Identity

Some scholars identify the phase of 'post-adolescence', that is, early 20s, as 'youth' or what Arnett (2000) has called 'emerging adulthood'. This is a critical phase of life, a period of major physical, physiological, psychological and behavioural changes with changing patterns of social interactions and relationships. Arnett (2000) considered this early 20s phase of 'emerging adulthood' as a period of individual volition, when young people explore different lifestyles, change residence more frequently than people in any other age group and experiment with intimate relationships and types of work and worldviews (Mortimer and Larson 2002).

Young people establish their own relationships and families, take on responsibility and agency and make key decisions not only for themselves but also for others who are closely linked to or dependent on them (Oliver and Pitt 2011). Being young they have the ability to learn faster and are more open to adopting new technologies, can innovate solutions and are also more flexible in adapting to different situations. Most enter the workforce, are economically productive and contribute to the economy at the family, community and national levels. They are also called on to play a larger role within the family and in social and political life and lead the process of continuity as well as change of social norms, values and mores in society (UNFPA 2014).

1.4 The Need to Focus on Adolescents and Youth in India

1.4.1 Demographic Significance

With 356 million young people aged 10–24 years, 253 million between the ages of 10 and 19 years and 231 million between 15 and 24 years, India has the largest number of adolescents and youth in the world. These young people comprise about 30% of the population (Census of India 2011). Every third person in the country is thus a 'young person', aged between 10 and 24 years (Census of India 2011). This is indeed a very substantial proportion of the population, and their needs and aspirations must be considered in national planning.

Globally, in 2012 there were around 1.6 billion young people aged 12–24 years who comprised almost a quarter of the world's population (United Nations 2012). Of this total number, 721 million were adolescents aged 12–17 and 850 million were youth aged 18–24 (United Nations 2012). While the growth of this cohort has reached its peak and is declining in most parts of the world, it is expected to rise in Africa till 2040 (United Nations 2012). India will continue to see this high proportion of adolescents and youth for the next two decades (Central Statistics Office, Ministry of Statistics and Programme Implementation 2017). In less than a decade from now, India, with a median age of 29 years, will be the youngest nation in the world (Kumar 2016; Patel 2013). It is therefore important to provide adequate attention to this cohort.

1.4.2 Demographic Dividend

The large cohort of young people in India represents a positive demographic outcome, resulting from the earlier higher, and now declining, birth rate. The ratio of dependent older persons as well as children to economically productive young persons is lower than if the birth rate had remained constant over the past few decades (UNFPA 2014). The higher proportion of economically and constructively contributing young adults thus provides a bonus, or demographic dividend, an opportunity for the economy and productivity to 'boom', or accelerate rapidly, due to the large share of productive young people contributing to its growth (UNFPA 2014).

India has a unique opportunity to ensure a brighter future by taking advantage of the demographic dividend of the large proportion of young people in the population. In order for persons in this cohort to realise their fullest potential, they must be healthy and well nourished, be appropriately educated and skilled and have access to opportunities for growth and productive engagement in work as well as in public life. Only then will the country be able to make substantial social, economic and environmental progress in the coming years.

1.4.3 Domain of Health and Fitness

Youth is the window of opportunity that sets the stage for a healthy and productive adulthood in later years (Sunitha and Gururaj 2014). Adult health is firmly based on the status of health as an adolescent and particularly influenced by adequate nurture during the growth spurt that marks this period. Cardiovascular fitness, muscular strength and body composition are at their peak during the late teens and early twenties and provide a good predictor of health and fitness later in life. Nearly 25% accrual of the bone mass of the skeletal system occurs in 2 years of rapid adolescent growth and can be influenced by nutrition and physical activity (Lancet Commission 2016). Similarly, brain and neural development continues well into the teens and early twenties. Responding to hormones that are released during adolescence, the neural system matures to handle emotions, awareness of the feelings and intentions of others and widening and diverse relationships and sociocultural complexities (Lancet Commission 2016).

Many of the habits and behaviours that affect the onset of non-communicable diseases are adopted at this stage in life, such as dietary and food consumption patterns; the use of tobacco, alcohol and psychotropic substances; and regular physical and mental activity. Similarly, positive coping mechanisms and positive psychosocial networks are also laid down at this time. The trajectory of future health is thus set in adolescence and young adulthood, and appropriate interventions at this stage can have long-range benefits.

Adolescence and youth are generally seen as a time of good health and well-being, but in reality there are several gaps that require attention. The causes of adolescent morbidity and mortality differ from those of younger children or older adults and often receive less attention. Further, these causes may lie outside the direct purview of the health sector – e.g. the leading cause of death among adolescent and young men is road accidents (Sivagurunathan et al. 2015), prevention of, and prompt attention to, which calls for multisectoral responses which health professionals often do not consider. For example, mental health of young people requires far more attention than is presently available given that 33% of police-reported suicides are among youth aged 18–30 years (Central Statistics Office, Government of India 2017). Moreover, adolescents are less likely to benefit from existing services because they are not perceived to be in need of these and have the lowest universal health coverage of any age group (Tylee et al. 2007). The unmet need for contraception is highest in this age group, as is the need to address unsafe abortions. Clearly young people face barriers to the use of services which result in compromised health as well as a weakened foundation for health in the future.

1.4.4 Diversity and Heterogeneity

Any attempt to focus on young people will require a nuanced understanding of the vast heterogeneity in this population across India. The situation, conditions and lives of adolescents and youth in India are extremely diverse, with different needs, life experiences, perspectives and aspirations, depending on geography, history, gender and socio-economic context. Starting with physical, mental and emotional growth, there are vast differences between adolescents, even those within the 5-year age range of subcategories. For instance, some adolescents reach puberty earlier, with marked changes in physical appearance as well sexual maturity, than others. Neurological as well as social development also occurs at different rates, as does the establishment of a sense of independence and self. Programmes for adolescents require flexibility to take cognisance of the different realities and needs of the diverse set of young people.

The differentiation is particularly striking for those residing in rural versus urban geographies, those from economically, educationally and socioculturally privileged backgrounds and those from less privileged and socially marginalised communities. There are vast differences in terms of access to health, education and prospects for growth and development and access to services and opportunities. The results of this diversity are apparent – for example, in terms of nutrition, young people face twin problems of undernutrition and stunting along with overnourishment and obesity (NIPCCD, New Delhi 2008).

1.5 Adolescence and Young Adults: The Present Scenario and the Gaps

Adolescence and youth are still not fully recognised as very important stages in development with their own peculiar needs and conditions. Adolescence especially is seen as merely an extension of childhood, and for young people only select sectors are addressed where they are viewed as part of a larger vulnerable group, e.g. promotion of livelihoods or prevention of ill health as in HIV-related activities or reproduction for young women. The special graded need for increased independence, agency, exploration and responsibility, or psychosocial well-being, is rarely acknowledged and accounted for. Programme design does not consider these needs adequately and most often considers them as being addressed through initiatives for children. More importantly, socially and legally adolescents are not considered able and therefore not empowered to make decisions regarding their own health and well-being. They are therefore prevented from taking positive action to seek health-care services and training courses and participate in social processes on their own initiative. This constrains their development and well-being. In many cases implementation of schemes and programmes aimed at the development of adolescents and youth does not cover the full country and is not sufficiently robust to bring about lasting change in the conditions, norms, values and customs that limit the fullest development of young people.

Overtime, there has been a considerable transformation in the lifestyles of the young due to increased urbanisation, individualisation and globalisation. This has resulted in problems related to nutrition, where malnutrition, obesity and eating disorders coexist; unsafe early onset sexual practices; psychosomatic disorders, such as depression, suicide and violence; and school dropout and substance abuse among school and college students and professionals working in urban and rural areas are increasing (NIPCCD, New Delhi 2008). All these, as well as many other issues related to adolescents and youth, need to be better studied and understood in order to design appropriate prevention and responsive services.

1.5.1 Rural-Urban Gap

Although there have been positive changes in the past few decades, there are large differences between the rural and urban scenarios. About two in five or 43% of the rural youth, as compared to 19% of urban youth, had not been to school (Populations Council and IIPS 2010). The opportunities available to both are qualitatively different; for example, the rural youth, who come to towns and cities in large numbers, have to struggle the hardest to access basic health and education services, jobs and livelihoods for themselves (UNFPA 2014). Women and rural adolescents continue to be at a greater disadvantage in terms of secondary and higher education (Census of India 2011). The inadequate food and residential arrangements, the overcrowding in educational institutions and the psychological tensions and insecurities generated by the more competitive, individualistic and impersonal environment of urban life, coupled with the uncertainties of future employment, result in inhibited socialisation of rural youth (Upadhyay 1995). Even within urban spaces, while some adolescents have access to the best education the world has to offer, others make do in dilapidated schools with no access to toilets, electricity or quality teachers. Some can pursue their dreams, while others must take on adult roles of earning and supporting the family while they are still minors and should be learning, growing and free from the burden of responsibility for others. Moreover, young people from marginalised communities, or with different sexual and gender orientations and preferences, face appalling stigma, discrimination and isolation, which deeply impacts their psychological health as well as learning outcomes (Ranade 2018). In a fast-changing world, the range of ambitions and demands of peers, parents, communities and society as well as their own aspirations place tremendous pressure on adolescents and youth of the new millennia, sometimes without the required opportunities, support and guidance to fulfil these multiple aspirations in a healthy manner. Better job opportunities and protection against crime and violence are similarly important to them. These responses show a lingering global need to provide the essential conditions for the full empowerment of young people. Young people see ‘a good education’, ‘better health care’ and ‘an honest and responsive government’ as actions that would make the greatest difference to their lives (UNICEF 2016).

1.5.2 Education/Training Gap

As mentioned, while there has been substantial progress in health and education, the progress is still uneven, and some young people are left behind. Enrolment in school is near universal, and India has reached its Millennium Development Goal, but school completion is still a distant goal. The mean years of schooling for India is 5.12 (Planning Commission Twelfth Five-Year Plan, 2012–2017 Govt. of India), lower than the average for developing countries, which is 7.09 years. Earlier, too, the Youth Study (International Institute for Population Sciences IIPS, Population Council 2010) found that just two in five young men and one in three young women had completed high school. For both young women and men, the main reason for dropping out is the need to take on an adult role – for girls, this is care of the household and children, and for boys it is the compulsion to earn. The same study found that over two-thirds of young men and one-half of young women had engaged in paid or unpaid work, at some point in their lives. Of these, over one in four young men and women had initiated work in early adolescence, before the age of 15. Adolescents and youth who are denied the opportunity to learn and explore different avenues cannot contribute their fullest to either their own or the country's future. This lack of schooling and early entry into the workforce and household sphere severely constrain building a foundation for continued education, training and better-paying work options. In addition, 27.5% of young people in India are not in employment, education or training and are virtually idle, with little to occupy them or to look forward to (World Bank 2012). This group is of special concern as they are readily recruited into disruptive activities and politicised for party gains and their frustrations channelised for causes they may not really understand or subscribe to. Instead of being the fountainhead of the future, these young people have a bleak future unless positive efforts to include them in development planning are made.

1.5.3 Gender Gap

The adolescent sex ratio has been low and was particularly low in 2001, at 882 females to 1000 males. This improved slightly to 898 (same as the 1961 level) in 2011, likely as a result of several interventions by national and state governments as well as civil society actors. Similarly, the youth sex ratio declined from 961 in 1971 to 939 in 2011 and is projected to fall to 904 by 2021 (Central Statistics Office 2017). The sex ratio clearly reflects the compromised position of females, son preference, and lack of nutrition and health care for the girl child. Moreover, the sex ratio is not uniform across the country but varies widely – from a low of 584 in the Union Territory of Daman and Diu to 1053 in Lakshadweep. Similarly, the youth sex ratio was 406 in Daman and Diu and 1040 in Puducherry. In terms of education, the National Youth Study (2006–2007) found that 47% of females and 26% of males had never been to school. In spite of the narrowing gender gap in school enrolment, young women continue to have very limited agency compared to young men, and adolescent boys and young men themselves have little agency. Studies on decision-making by adolescents showed that while both girls and boys can decide who to make friends with, they are less likely to make decisions regarding spending money or buying their own clothes. Only one in four young women made decisions in all three areas, according to the Youth Study, and about 56% of young men made these decisions. Similarly, the mobility of girls and young women is more restricted than that of young men, but more than one-third of young men were not permitted to attend programmes or entertainment outside their village or neighbourhood or to visit a health facility unescorted. While more young women than men had money saved fewer had a bank account, and of those who did, 54% operated the account themselves, as against 90% of young men. Although adolescents and youth are viewed as the pioneers of change and as displaying more egalitarian values, their attitudes to gender, a critical aspect for India, are inconsistent and not well integrated. Thus while most adolescent girls and boys agree that educating girls is as important as educating boys and that girls are as good as boys in studies, over half of all adolescents (52% girls and 56% boys and 58% young women and 54% young men) felt husbands are justified in beating their wives in at least one situation. Further, although the government and civil society organisations now organise several programmes for adolescents and young people, only 22% of young men and 31% of young women were aware of these programmes, and only 12% of young men and 9% of young women reported they had participated in such programmes. While there was no data on adolescent participation, given that adolescents have less mobility and are not allowed to even access health facilities on their own, it is likely that participation is even more limited (IIPS and Population Council 2010).

Available data clearly indicates that while there is potential for reaping a high productive gain from the demographic dividend, and there has been substantial progress on several indicators, adolescents and young people face serious challenges in making the transition to healthy, responsible adulthood, equipped with skills and education to blossom and achieve their aspirations. These challenges lie largely in the family, community and larger sociocultural and legal framework that defines this stage of life, and at present adolescents and young people have little space or recognition to take the steps required to walk confidently towards adulthood. Appropriate policies, programmes and interventions with key gatekeepers and stakeholders will be effective to change the present paradigm and ensure a brighter future.

1.6 Investing in Young People

1.6.1 Benefits of Investing in Young People

The fruits of this excellent opportunity to reap a rich demographic dividend from the large potential workforce can be realised only through well-informed strategic investment in adolescents and youth. Recent studies (Sheehan et al. 2017) clearly establish the benefits of investing in young people. Investments in adolescents and youth have a triple return or dividend – they result in better health, well-being and capability for the present generation of young people; produce healthy, responsible and constructive adults in the near future; and provide an intergenerational return in terms of the health and well-being of the next generation of children, born to these young people (Lancet Commission 2016). Well-integrated and thoughtfully designed investments in the health and well-being of adolescents provide high economic and social returns as lives saved, morbidity and injury averted, better control over fertility, improved human capital and improved relationships in families and communities translate into increased and improved labour supply, employment, productivity, job quality and capital. These investments also lead to an enhanced position of women in families and communities and stronger communities (Sheehan et al. 2017). The present cohort of young people is seen as critical in achieving the Sustainable Development Goals (SDGs), as they can take forward emerging ideas of holistic development and implement programmes that protect the environment, conserve and renew resources and build strong, interconnected, equitable communities and nations. Adolescents and youth are, therefore, the foundation of the future, and appropriate and adequate policies and programmes for them are an essential development priority for all countries. A better understanding of the structural and social determinants of health and well-being indicates that these investments need to go far beyond narrow sectoral efforts in the traditional youth-related sectors such as education, sports, health and skills development. A focus on adolescents and youth is thus essential not only because they constitute a major portion of the population and that this section of the population is the most productive and can drive the economy as well as governance to rich returns but also because their well-being requires attention. Appropriate investments in their health and well-being are essential to provide healthy adults and parents for the next generation and a brighter future for the country. However, investing in individual adolescents and youth without changing the context and the structure of laws, policies and social norms is unlikely to produce the macro impact desired. This aspect has been discussed in the following section.

1.6.2 The Importance of Laws and Policies

Young people benefit greatly from structural interventions and supportive laws. For example, raising the legal age of marriage and therefore of child-bearing impacts positively on the sexual and reproductive health of women and also on their overall health, both mental and physical. Coupled with compulsory schooling and the right to education, girls have access to education, training and skills, have the opportunity to be independent and more productive economically, participate more fully in civic affairs and live more healthy fulfilling lives. Similarly, labour laws that restrict the hiring of minors increase the period of schooling for adolescent boys and expand their world of possibilities. The regulation of work in hazardous occupations serves to protect young workers. Simple measures such as the compulsory use of helmets while riding two wheelers can reduce death rates from road accidents among this age group significantly (Lancet Commission 2016). At the same time, some laws that seek to 'protect' adolescents can have a negative impact. For instance, the need for parental/guardian consent for abortions or access to some forms of long-acting contraception proves to be a major barrier for young people who are extremely sensitive and fear stigma greatly. They are then pushed into the use of unregulated, unsafe health services which can have long-lasting negative impacts on their health, and even cause death.

In the past few decades, a number of policies, schemes and programmes have been launched by the Indian government with the aim of holistic development of adolescents and youth, to enable them to achieve their full potential (Kumar et al. 2012). These have been mainly through central and state schemes related to education, nutrition, sexual and reproductive health, empowerment of girl children and changing social norms and customs that restrict the growth and development of particularly girls.

The considerable investments in mainly education and health have produced positive results, and the 2011 census indicates that literacy and enrolment in higher education have improved significantly (Census of India 2011). The prevalence rates of some communicable diseases among young people have decreased, largely due to effective immunisation campaigns. The use of tobacco by young people is also less common than before, likely due to widespread education and publicity about the negative effects of tobacco on health among youth in India (Chandrupatla et al. 2017).

The National Youth Policy 2014 is aimed at 15–29-year-olds and envisions to 'empower the youth of the country to achieve their full potential, and through them, enable India to find its rightful place in the community of nations' (National Youth Policy 2014, Govt. of India). Five objectives have been defined, with action called for in 11 priority areas. The objectives are to (1) create a productive workforce; (2) develop a strong and healthy generation; (3) instil social values and promote community service; (4) facilitate participation and civic engagement; and (5) support youth at risk and create equitable opportunities for all. The vision spelled out in the National Youth Policy presents a good opportunity to revisit and review our approach to young people. India will continue to have a very large proportion of young people with a median age of 28 for another decade and will thus have a massive workforce of 592 million in 2020 (NYP, Govt. of India 2014), which can power impressive economic growth. Also, as India aspires to move towards greater development, its aspirations and goals are moving from the margins and 'emergency' responses to very severe problems to consolidating development and a more proactive, positive response. It is now ready to look beyond the prevention of mortality to health and well-being and beyond handling immediate crises to investing in the future. Part of this new-found confidence is being channelled into investing in adolescents and youth. The Government of India (GoI) currently invests more than Rs 90,000 crores per annum, 37,000 crores through youth-targeted (higher education, skill development, health care, etc.) and 55,000 crores through nontargeted schemes designed for various demographic segments of which youth are significant beneficiaries such as food subsidies and employment programmes. This works out to approximately Rs 2710 per young individual per year (Union Budget 2011–2012). This is a significant amount and if invested wisely can make a difference not only in the individual lives of adolescents and young people but for the future of the country. Social media and access to the Internet and to mobile smartphones have opened a whole new world to young people. Their sources of information and willingness to 'chat' and thereby connect with persons from different backgrounds create ways of peer interaction and learning that could not be imagined before. These are likely very positive avenues of broadening horizons, and their potential for reaching adolescents can be further explored and strengthened. This is indeed an ambitious and holistic vision and requires all stakeholders to align and collaborate for its realisation.

Some other significant legal instruments that form the basis for the empowerment of young people are the Right to Education Act, 2010; the Prohibition of Child Marriage Act, 2006; Child Labour Act, 1986; and the Protection of Children from Sexual Offences Act, 2012. While all of these are motivated by a laudable intent to address key aspects of young people's growth and development, investing in enhancing young people's capabilities is not accorded the required emphasis and priority. As a result the desired goal is yet to be fully achieved.

This Volume: Bridging the Information Gap

Recognising the urgency of the need to focus greater and more meaningful attention on adolescents and youth as well as identify the gaps in information and understanding, Tata Institute of Social Sciences and UNFPA collaborated on a Centre of Excellence on Adolescents and Youth. The centre undertook extensive reviews of the situation of young people through desk reviews in four streams: nutrition, sexual and reproductive health, mental health and livelihoods and social entrepreneurship. The reviews were complemented by consultations with experts in each thematic area, individually as well as in groups. The work on each thematic area forms the chapters of this volume. Each chapter covers the following:

- An overview of the present situation of adolescents and young people in the selected stream, viz. nutrition, sexual and reproductive health including HIV and AIDS, mental health and livelihoods.
- Identification of gaps in information and in research.
- A review of policies and programmes for young people.
- A critique of policies and programmes, including the identification of initiatives that have been particularly effective.
- A summary of key issues and recommendations that must be considered in designing policies and programmes for young people for the future.

During the review process and through interactions with experts on adolescents and youth, the need for developing capacity in undertaking research on adolescents and youth emerged strongly. A qualitative study on evaluating capacity for research with adolescents and youth was thus undertaken, and the result forms the last chapter of this volume.

We see this book as contributing to the body of work on adolescents and youth at a very opportune time, when there is a growing urgency to address their needs and thus strengthen the foundation for sustainable development. As it brings together reviews of research as well as policy and programmes, it will be of interest to scholars and researchers, policymakers and planners, as well as to all those interested in young people. We hope it will draw more attention to young people, stimulate discussion and engage adolescents and youth in the dialogue on their future.

References

Apter, T. (2013). *Difficult mothers: Understanding and overcoming their power*. New York: Norton & Company.

Arnett, J. (2000). Emerging adulthood: A theory of development from late teens through the twenties. *American Psychologist, 55*(5), 469–480.

Census of India. (2011). *Age data*. http://www.censusindia.gov.in/2011census/population_enumeration.html. Accessed 14 Apr 2017.

Central Statistics Office. (2017). *Statistical year book India 2017*. Ministry of Statistics and Programme Implementation Government of India (Social Statistics Division). http://www.mospi.gov.in/statistical-year-book-india/2017. Accessed 12 Apr 2017.

Chandrupatla, S. G., Tavares, M., & Natto, Z. S. (2017). Tobacco use and effects of professional advice on smoking cessation among youth in India. *Asian Pacific Journal of Cancer Prevention, 18*(7), 1861–1867. https://doi.org/10.22034/APJCP.2017.18.7.1861.

Chaudhary, N., & Sharma, N. (2012). In J. J. Arnett (Ed.), *Adolescent psychology around the world* (pp. 113–118). New York: Psychology Press.

Erikson, E. H. (1959). Identity and the life cycle. *Psychological Issues, 1*, 1–171.

International Institute for Population Sciences (IIPS) and Population Council. (2010). *Youth in India: Situations and needs 2006–2007*. Mumbai: IIPS. http://iipsindia.org/pdf/India%20 Report.pdf. Accessed 24 April 2017.

Jain, M. (2014). Sabla: The road to empowerment and self esteem for adolescent girls. *Yojana, 58*(January), 63–64.

Johnson, S. B., Blum, R. W., & Giedd, J. N. (2009). Adolescent maturity and the brain: The promise and pitfalls of neuroscience research in adolescent health policy. *Journal of Adolescent Health, 45*, 216–221.

Kumar, S. (2016). The time of youth. *Economic & Political Weekly, 51*(53), 102–109.

Kumar, A. S., Labeeb, M. P. K., Abraham, S. S., & Mathai, S. M. (2012). Issues in holistic development of adolescents. In *Handbook of management and behavioural science* (Vol. VI). Delhi: Wisdom publications.

Lancet Commission. (2016). *Our future: A Lancet commission on adolescent health and wellbeing*. https://www.thelancet.com/commissions/adolescent-health-and-wellbeing. Accessed 11 Mar 2017.

Lerner, R. M. (Ed.). (1993). *Early adolescence: Perspectives on research, policy, and intervention*. Hillsdale: Erlbaum.

Ministry of Youth Affairs and Sports (MoYAS). (2014). *National youth policy 2014*. New Delhi: MoYAS, Government of India.

Mortimer, J. T., & Larson, R. W. (2002). Macrostructural trends and the reshaping of adolescence. In J. T. Mortimer & R. W. Larson (Eds.), *The changing adolescent experience: Societal trends and the transition to adulthood*. Cambridge: Cambridge University Press.

National Institute of Public Cooperation and Child Development (NIPCCD), New Delhi. (2008). *Studies on adolescent girls: An analytical review*. http://nipccd.nic.in/reports/eag.pdf. Accessed 15 Mar 2017.

Oliver, B., & Pitt, B. (Eds.). (2011). *Working with children, young people and families: A course book for foundation degrees*. London: Sage.

Patel, V. (2013). Indian youth at the crossroads. *Indian Journal of Human Development, 7*(1), 193–204.

Planning Commission of India. (2013). *Twelfth five year plan 2007–12, Volume II (Social Sector)*. New Delhi: Sage. http://planningcommission.gov.in/plans/planrel/12thplan/pdf/12fyp_vol3.pdf. Accessed 11 Mar 2017.

Ranade, K. (2018). *Growing up gay in urban India: A critical psychosocial perspective*. Singapore: Springer.

Saraswathi, T. S. (1999). Adult-child continuity in India: Is adolescence a myth or an emerging reality? In T. S. Saraswathi (Ed.), *Culture, socialization and human development* (pp. 214–232). New Delhi: Sage.

Saraswathi, T. S., & Dutta, R. (1988). *Invisible boundaries: Grooming for adult roles*. New Delhi: Northern Book Centre.

Saraswathi, T. S., & Oke, M. (2013). Ecology of adolescence in India: Implications for policy and practice. *Psychological Studies, 58*(4), 353–364.

Schlegel, A., & Barry, H., III. (1991). *Adolescence: An anthropological inquiry*. New York: Free Press.

Sheehan, P., Sweeny, K., Rasmussen, B., et al. (2017). Building the foundations for sustainable development: A case for global investment in the capabilities of adolescents. *Lancet, 390*(10104), 1792–1806. https://doi.org/10.1016/S0140-6736(17)30872-3.

Sivagurunathan, C., Umadevi, R., Rama, R., & Gopalakrishnan, S. (2015). Adolescent health: Present status and its related Programmes in India. Are we in the right direction? *Journal of Clinical and Diagnostic Research, 9*(3), LE01–LE06.

Stang, J., & Story, M. (2005). Adolescent growth and development. In *Guidelines for adolescent nutrition services*. Minneapolis, MN Center for Leadership, Education and Training in Maternal and Child Nutrition, Division of Epidemiology and Community Health, School of Public Health, University of Minnesota; 2005. http://www.epi.umn.edu/let/pubs/img/adol_ch1.pdf. Accessed 17 Mar 2017.

Sunitha, S., & Gururaj, G. (2014). Health behaviours & problems among young people in India: Cause for concern & call for action. *Indian Journal of Medical Research, 140*(2), 185.

Tylee, A., Haller, D. M., Graham, T., Churchill, R., & Sanci, L. A. (2007). Youth-friendly primary-care services: How are we doing and what more needs to be done? *Lancet, 369*, 1565–1573.

UNICEF (2016). *My world survey 2015*. Available from: https://www.unngls.org/IMG/pdf/MY_World_Report_Monrovia.pdf. Accessed 11 Apr 2017.

United Nations. (2012). *World population prospects, the 2012 revision*. http://www.un.org/en/development/desa/publications/world-population-prospects-the-2012-revision.html. Accessed 08 Apr 2017.

United Nations Population Fund (UNFPA). (2014). *Annual report: A year of renewal*. http://www.unfpa.org/annual-report-2014. Accessed 10 Mar 2017.

United Nations Population Fund (UNFPA). (2015). *For people, planet and prosperity*. https://www.unfpa.org/sites/default/files/pub-pdf/UNFPA_2015_Annual_Report.pdf. Accessed 10 Mar 2017.

Upadhyay, H. C. (1995). Youth in the Indian society: With special reference to rural youth. In N. Mohammad & A. Matin (Eds.), *Indian youth: Problems and prospects*. New Delhi: Ashish Publishing House.

Verma, S., & Saraswathi, T. S. (2002). Adolescents in India: Street Urchins or Silicon Valley Millionnaires? In R. Larson & T. S. Saraswathi (Eds.), *The world's youth: Adolescence in eight regions of the globe*. New York: Cambridge University Press.

Way, A. (2014). *USAID youth data collection in DHS surveys: An overview*. (Paper no. 9).

World Bank. (2012). *World development report 2012: Gender equality and development*. https://openknowledge.worldbank.org/handle/10986/4391. Accessed 12 Apr 2017.

Chapter 2
Adolescent and Youth Nutrition in India

Hemal Shroff and Deepa Shokeen

Abstract This chapter is a comprehensive review of the current status of nutrition among adolescents and youth in India. It presents contemporary literature on the prevalence of underweight, overweight and obesity among these subpopulations and highlights areas where there is inadequate data. The prevalence of micronutrient deficiencies among Indian adolescents and youth, as well as among specific vulnerable populations, is also briefly described. Policies and programmes that have a direct or indirect impact on nutrition are described in detail along with reviews of their impact, where evidence is available. The review also includes a section on vulnerable populations and discusses factors that affect dietary intake and nutrition, including knowledge levels among adolescents and youth. Recommendations for policy-level, programmatic, community-level and research initiatives to improve nutrition and fill the gaps in research are made with a view to highlighting the important issue of nutrition among this relatively neglected demographic sub-group in India.

Keywords Underweight · Micronutrient deficiency · National nutrition policy · Nutrition programmes · Overweight

2.1 Introduction

The terms 'adolescence', 'young adults', 'youth' and 'emerging adults' are variably used to define adolescents and youth across multiple settings. In general, these terms refer to individuals between the ages of 10 and 15 (adolescents) and 15 and 24 years (youth), which is based on definitions used by the World Health Organisation and other UN organisations (WHO 2005; UNFPA 2003; UN DESA 2004). Adolescence is a critical period of growth and development. In this period, humans go through the second biggest growth spurt of their lives (after the first 5 years of life). Adolescents, both girls and boys, are particularly vulnerable to the effects of

H. Shroff (✉) · D. Shokeen
Centre for Excellence on Adolescents & Youth, Tata Institute of Social Sciences, Mumbai, India

S. Bharat, G. Sethi (eds.), *Health and Wellbeing of India's Young People*,
https://doi.org/10.1007/978-981-13-6593-5_2

undernutrition. For boys and girls, it is the time when the body readies itself for the physical demands of being a part of the adult workforce. For girls, it is also the time when the body prepares itself for the nutritional demands of pregnancy and lactation that they will soon experience. Physiologically, nutritional status in adolescence is strongly connected with risk for several diseases later in life. Behaviourally, food choices and unhealthy eating habits in adolescence and young adulthood tend to be continued into middle adulthood and later in life. Thus, nutrition among adolescents and youth is a crucial area of research and intervention (Box 2.1).

Box 2.1 Definitions of Terms Used to Describe the Nutritional Status of Adolescents and Youth

Undernutrition is defined as being underweight for one's age, too short for one's age (stunted), dangerously thin for one's height (wasted) and deficient in vitamins and minerals (micronutrient malnutrition) (UNICEF 2006).

Protein energy malnutrition (PEM) is a condition where there is inadequate protein or caloric intake.

Underweight/thinness, as per WHO-BMI for age criteria is the condition where the *Z* score for BMI for age falls between one and two standard deviations (SD) below the median. Thinness can be used as a proxy indicator for undernutrition as defined by weight-for-age criteria, which has limited value among adolescents.

Severe thinness is defined as less than two standard deviations below the WHO growth standard median.

Overweight is defined as a BMI greater than 1 SD above the WHO growth standard median for children and adolescents (age 5–19 years). For Asian adults (> 18 years), overweight is defined as a BMI greater than or equal to 23.

Obesity is defined for children and adolescents (ages 5–19 years) as a BMI that is more than 2 SD above the WHO growth standard median. For Asian adults (> 18 years), obesity is defined as a body mass index (BMI) greater than or equal to 25.

Of about 1.8 billion young people in the world, 356 million, i.e. the highest, are residing in India (UNFPA 2014), thus making them a crucial demographic to focus efforts on. It is essential to meet the needs of young people as they have the potential to contribute significantly to the economic and social progress of India. By investing in adolescent and youth nutrition, there are significant short- and long-term economic benefits as well as other advantages, e.g. better health for future generations, large savings in health costs, better education, increased intellectual capacity and greater well-being (United Nations Administrative Committee on Coordination/Sub-committee on Nutrition 2000). The cycle of nutrition (as well as malnutrition) impacts not just the current generation but future generations as well. In addition, from a rights perspective, having access to adequate food for optimal growth should be a fundamental right for all Indian adolescents and youth. In the next few years, India has a unique opportunity in the form of its demographic dividend (i.e. the heightened development that can occur when a substantial percentage of the population is of working age), which makes it all the more crucial to focus on adolescents and youth, as they are the future workforce of the country and the world. And yet, there is little that has been done to improve the nutrition and health of this section of the population. This chapter focuses on adolescent and youth nutrition in India, highlighting the current nutritional status, factors affecting nutritional status, deficiencies, programmes and policies, gaps in research with proposed recommendations and strategies to combat nutrition deficiencies among this underserved section of the population.

2.2 Prevalence

2.2.1 The Prevalence of Underweight Among Adolescents and Youth in India

India's progress towards the Sustainable Development Goals (SDG's 2, 3 and 6) is off-track due to the persistence of underweight among children and adolescents and the dual burden of undernutrition and overweight among adult populations. More than one-fifth of adults are too thin, and a little less than 20% are overweight or obese in India (IIPS 2016). Only 61% of men and 57% of women (including young adults) are at a healthy weight for their height (IIPS/Macro International 2007). Based on the National Family Health Survey Fourth round (NFHS-4) data, the prevalence of undernutrition is higher in rural adults, both males (23%) and females (26.7%) in comparison to urban males (15.3%) and females (15.5%) (IIPS 2016). Overall, the variation between undernutrition among adults in urban and rural areas has reduced drastically when comparing the NFHS-4 with the NFHS-3 results. However, these figures highlight the critical situation of the nutrition status of young people in India, as both conditions of underweight and overweight put people at risk for illness and a suboptimal quality of life (see Table 2.1).

According to a National Nutrition Monitoring Bureau (NNMB 2012) survey done in the rural areas of 12 states of India, the overall prevalence of thinness among 10–13-year boys was about 47%, and severe thinness was 18%, while in girls, it was 36% and 12%, respectively. Among boys of 14–17 years of age, the overall prevalence of thinness was about 41%, and severe thinness was 16%, while in girls of the same age, it was 23% and 6%, respectively. UNICEF's most recent report on adolescents states that nearly 50% of Indian adolescent girls (15–19 years) are underweight, with a body mass index of less than 18.5 (2012). According to the NFHS-3 findings, compared to adolescent boys, adolescent girls in India have lower levels of nutrition, poorer access to adequate, healthy food and requisite healthcare (IIPS/Macro International 2007). The differences in the sex distribution of underweight are a result of the differences in the samples for the various surveys. There are substantial differences in prevalence of underweight between adolescents and young adults across the various states of the country and even within states.

Table 2.1 Prevalence of Undernutrition[a] among adolescents in India (10–19 years)

S.No	Author	Year and region	Age group (years)	Undernutrition[a] prevalence %		
				Boys	Girls	Overall
1.	Wasnik et al.	2012, Andhra Pradesh	10–15	–	Underweight – 56.4	56.4
2.	Maliye et al.	2010, Wardha, Maharashtra	10–19	–	Thin – 57	57
3.	Jeemon et al.	2009, India	10–19	–	–	Underweight – 53.2
4.	Haboubi & Shaikh	2009, Tamil Nadu	10–16	Stunted – 38.8 thin – 64.6	Stunted – 36.9 Thin – 50.1	–
5.	Laxmaiah et al.	2007, Andhra Pradesh	12–17	Undernourished – 45	Undernourished – 21	–
6.	Deshmukh et al.	2006, Wardha, Maharashtra	10–19	–	–	Thin – 53.8 Wasted – 20.8
7.	Rao et al.	2003, Madhya Pradesh	1119	–	–	Underweight – 61.7 Stunted – 51.7 Wasted – 32.8

[a]Various cut-offs used

Studies done among underserved and vulnerable populations suggest a more critical situation. Rao and Vijay (2006) conducted studies on tribal populations in Bihar, which revealed higher than average prevalence of undernutrition. Balgir et al. (2002) assessed the health and nutritional status of Gond children in the Kalahandi district of Orissa and found that 89.3% of the children and adolescents between the ages of 6 and 14 years were underweight. Chakrabarty and Bharati (2010) investigated the nutritional status among Shabar children (5–19 years) living in urban, rural and forest habitats and the factors associated with their nutritional status. Among these children, those from the forest regions had the highest prevalence of undernutrition (33.87%) followed by their rural (24.62%) and urban counterparts (20.16%), respectively. It is hypothesised that insufficient food, along with traditional sociocultural and physical activities, may lead to a high proportion of tribal child as well as adult undernutrition (Balgir et al. 2002; Rao et al. 2007a, b; Banik 2009). Higher prevalence of malaria in the forest areas might also contribute to increased stunting and underweight among children and adolescents.

Protein energy malnutrition (PEM) is one other indicator of poor nutrition status. The table below (Table 2.2) presents the data on PEM among male and female adolescents of various age groups from rural parts of India (NNMB 2012). It is evident from the table that protein and calorie inadequacy ranged from 11.4% to 21.5%. On the other hand, protein-calorie adequacy ranged from 20.0% to 70.7% among adolescents and young adults. Across all age groups, calorie inadequacy

Table 2.2 Protein-calorie adequacy percentages (based on NNMB Survey 2012)

Age category	n	P- C-	P+ C-	P+ C+	P- C+
Boys (10–12 years)	1654	11.4	47.8	40.7	–
Girls (10–12 years)	1577	14.3	42.6	43.1	–
Boys (13–15 years)	1529	18.4	54.5	27.1	–
Girls (13–15 years)	1538	21.3	38.8	39.9	–
Boys (16–17 years)	898	21.2	50.9	20.0	–
Girls (16–17 years)	991	21.5	36.3	42.2	–
Adult men (sedentary)	4774	18.0	17.9	63.4	0.7
Adult women (sedentary)	9519	16.4	10.4	70.7	2.4

Note: *P+* protein adequate, *P-* protein inadequate, *C+* calorie adequate, *C-* calorie inadequate

appears to be a bigger problem than protein inadequacy. However, PEM continues to place a significant burden on adolescent and youth growth and development. Poor access to food and inadequate knowledge about dietary requirements are the common causes of PEM. Adolescents and young adults were classified as consuming inadequate amounts of calories and protein based on the age-appropriate recommended dietary intake for Indians (Table 2.3).

2.2.2 *Prevalence of Overweight and Obesity Among Adolescents and Youth*

India is a vast and diverse country with substantial variation in overweight and obesity across the states (Pednekar 2008). Research studies among adolescents from different parts of India like Delhi, Maharashtra, Punjab and South India include prevalence rates of overweight and obesity from 11% all the way to 29% (Kotian et al. 2010; Stigler 2011; Gupta et al. 2011; Raj 2009; Bharati et al. 2008). The percentage of overweight and obese children and adolescents has also been increasing in India. Based on data from the NFHS-3 (IIPS 2005) and NFHS-4 (IIPS 2016), the percentage of boys and men between the ages of 15 and 49 who are overweight or obese has doubled from 9.3% to 18.6% between these two rounds of the survey. The increase in value for girls and women for the same time period is close to double as well (12.6–20.7%). While most studies use measurements of height and weight to assess overweight and obesity, research indicates that Indians, while appearing thin, have higher body fat volumes than Caucasians, African Americans and other ethnic groups (Banerji et al. 1999), which places them at higher risk for diabetes and coronary heart disease. Thus, it is necessary to measure overweight and obesity in a more detailed manner in future research (Poobalan and Aucott 2016). The most important consequence of obesity in adolescence is its persistence into adulthood with associated health risks like cardiovascular diseases, diabetes, osteoarthritis, gallbladder disease, etc. Obesity is more likely to persist when its onset is in late childhood or adolescence.

Table 2.3 Prevalence of overweight/obesity[b] among adolescents in India

S. No	Author	Year and region	Age group	Overweight prevalence[b] %			Obesity prevalence[b] %		
				Boys	Girls	Overall	Boys	Girls	Overall
1.	Kapil et al.	2002, New Delhi	10–16	23.1	27.7	24.7	8.3	5.5	7.4
2.	Ramachandran et al.	2002, Chennai	13–18	17.8	15.8	–	3.6	2.9	–
3.	Chhatwal et al.	2004, Punjab	9–15	15.7	2.9	–	12.4	9.9	–
4.	Sidhu et al.	2005, Punjab	10–15	9.9	12.0	10.9	5.0	6.3	5.6
5.	Gupta et al.	2006, Jaipur	11–17	–	10.9	10.9	–	5.5	5.5
6.	Rao et al.	2007a, b, Pune	9–16	27.5	20.9	–		–	–
7.	Bhardwaj et al.	2008, New Delhi	14–17	–	–	–	–	–	24.3[a]
8.	Gupta et al	2011, New Delhi	14–17	–	–	25.2	–	–	11.7
9.	Nawab et al.	2014, UP	10–16	–	–	9.8	–	–	4.8
10.	Jagadesan et al.	2014, Chennai	6–17	20.7[a]	21.3[a]	–	–	–	–
11.	Chaitali et al.	2014, Bangalore	6–17	54.4	45.6	–	65.8	34.2	–

Note: [a]Overweight/obesity; [b]Various cut-offs used

Thus, just as reported for undernutrition, the statistics on overweight and obesity indicate substantial disparity across different parts of the country and between boys and girls. In general, rates of overweight are higher among higher socioeconomic groups, adolescents in private schools, in more developed states and among those in urban areas. Notably, there is little separate data on overweight and obesity among youth, especially those between the ages of 18 and 24.

There are few large-scale studies on the causes for the increasing prevalence of overweight and obesity in India. Some authors suggest that the same causal factors (sedentary lifestyles, increase in caloric consumption) apply in developing countries as are applicable for high rates of overweight and obesity in developed countries; however, there is inadequate research to support these assumptions. In addition, structural factors (such as access to public spaces for engaging in physical activity, affordability and accessibility of healthy foods, advertising of processed and unhealthy foods) that contribute to lower physical activity and unhealthy food consumption do not get investigated or targeted in interventions. Additionally, Indian adolescents and youth are increasingly exposed to foods that are made by multinational food companies, many of which are unhealthy, and this needs to be studied further. Thus, there is a dearth of research on etiological factors for overweight and obesity, as well as changing trends in rates of overweight and obesity among emerging adults (see Table 2.4).

Table 2.4 Studies on micronutrient deficiencies among Indian adolescent and youth populations

Author	Year and region	Age	Micronutrient deficiencies								
			Anaemia/ iron def./ ferritin (%)	Folic scid (%)	Vit. B12 (%)	Vit. A (%)	Vit. B complex (%)	Vit. C (%)	Zinc Def. (%)	Vit. D (% deficient)	Iodine (%)
Agarwal et al.	2003, Delhi	11–18	A – 49.3 Fe – 85	–	–	–	–	–	–	–	–
Marwaha et al.	2005, Delhi	10–18	–	–	–	–	–	–	–	LIG – 92.6 HIG – 84.9	–
Toteja et al.	2006, Multi centric	11–18	A – 90.1	–	–	–	–	–	–	–	–
Thankachan et al.	2007, Bangalore	18–35	A – 30 Fe – 62	–	–	–	–	–	–	–	–
Sethy et al.	2007, Orissa	6–12	–	–	–	–	–	–	–	–	Goitre – 23.6
Harinarayan	2007, Andhra Pradesh	Young adults and adults	–	–	–	–	–	–	–	Rural (M – 44, F – 7); Urban(M – 62, F – 75)	–
Puri et al.	2008, Delhi	6–18	–	–	–	–	–	–	–	11.5	–
Kapil et al.	2011, Delhi	11–18	–	–	–	–	–	–	49.4	-	–
Menon et al.	2011, Multicentric	18–30	Fe-66	2	34	4	–	–	52	-	–
Marwaha et al.	2011, Delhi	College girls	–	–	–	–	–	–	–	100	–
Unnikrishnan et al	2013, Multicentric	18–35	–	–	–	–	–	–	–	–	7.53 (Hyperthyroidism)
Chaudhary et al.	2013, Punjab	6–12	–	–	–	–	–	–	–	–	Goitre – 12.6

(continued)

Table 2.4 (continued

Author	Year and region	Age	Micronutrient deficiencies								
			Anaemia/ iron def./ ferritin (%)	Folic scid (%)	Vit. B12 (%)	Vit. A (%)	Vit. B complex (%)	Vit. C (%)	Zinc Def. (%)	Vit. D (% deficient)	Iodine (%)
Agarwal, Agarwal & Dharamendra	2013, UP	0–15	A – 11.8	–	–	Xerophthalmia – 5.4	–	–	–	–	–
Krishna & Mishra	2013, UP	11–18	–	–	–	1.25	14.8	10.5	–	–	–
Garg et al	2013, Delhi	Adolescents	–	–	–	–	–	–	–	96.9	–
Bhambhani, Bhambhani & Thakor	2015	10–19	Fe – 62.7	–	–	6.3	16.5	10	–	–	–
Bansal et al.	2016, Delhi	11–18	A – 58.7; SF – 41.1	5	63.3	–	–	–	–	–	–

2.2.3 Prevalence of Micronutrient Deficiencies

Due to increasing nutritional demands as a result of age-related rapid growth and development, adolescents are more susceptible to long-term micronutrient deficiencies (MNDs), if their diet is nutritionally inadequate. The most common micronutrients where there are deficiencies include vitamin A, folate, iron, iodine, vitamin B complex, vitamin D and Zinc. Coexistence of multiple micronutrient deficiencies (multiple MNDs) frequently occurs, especially in vulnerable groups like pregnant women and adolescents. MNDs occur due to insufficient dietary intake or sufficient intake coupled with impaired absorption of food due to infections, diseases and other inflammatory conditions (UNICEF 2013; Katona and Katona-Apte 2008). As is apparent from the table below, there are few large-scale studies on MNDs among adolescents and even fewer among youth. In many cases, data collected on dietary recall is used to provide evidence for inadequate consumption of vitamins and minerals. In a large-scale study across rural areas of several states, the National Nutrition Monitoring Bureau (NNMB) reported on the dietary intake of individuals across different age groups (NNMB 2012). There was a decline in consumption of foods rich in calcium, vitamin A, folate and iron for boys between the ages of 10 and 17 between 1996–1997 and 2011–2012. Similarly, for girls of the same age groups, there was a decline in consumption of foods high in iron, calcium and vitamin A for the same time period.

2.2.3.1 Vitamin A Deficiency (VAD)

According to the WHO (2009), 85% of South Asian children with xerophthalmia (a symptom of VAD) reside in India, and a significant increase has been reported in the prevalence of VAD among Indian women from 2001 (5.9%) to 2011 (30.3%). Very little research on vitamin A has been done in older children, adolescents and adults. VAD usually clusters within families, and it can be assumed that vitamin A status in other life stages is low in places where VAD is more prevalent in pregnant women (WHO 2009), which is suggestive of in utero influences.

2.2.3.2 Iron Deficiency

Iron deficiency has been and continues to be one of India's major public health problems. Consequences of iron deficiency are nutritional anaemia and lower resistance to infection (Welch 2002). In addition, anaemia and iron deficiency affect pregnant and lactating women, resulting in adverse pregnancy outcomes, such as low birth weight, still birth and impaired mental, physical and cognitive performance in children, and it is a significant risk factor for maternal mortality. Anaemia during adolescence has been linked with decreased physical and mental capacity, lesser ability to concentrate at work, poorer educational performance, poorer attention

Table 2.5 Prevalence of anaemia among women and men aged 15–24 years (NFHS-3)

		Women (%)		Men (%)	
S. No	Types of anaemia	15–19 years	20–24 years	15–19 years	20–24 years
1	Mild	39.1	38.2	16.7	10.5
2	Moderate	14.9	16.6	12.1	7.3
3	Severe	1.7	1.8	1.4	1.1
4	Any anaemia	55.7	56.7	30.2	19.0

span, memory loss, higher school dropout rate, stunted growth, increased susceptibility to infections and weakened immunity, delay in onset of menarche and irregularities in menstruation if already attained (WHO 2001).

According to the NFHS-4 findings, 53% of women and 22.7% of men aged 15–24 years are anaemic (IIPS 2015). From the NFHS-3, it was reported that adolescent girls (15–19 years) and young women aged 20–24 are equally likely to be anaemic (see Table 2.5), while the prevalence of anaemia among adolescent boys (15–19 years) is more (30.2%) in comparison to young men aged 20–24 years (19%) (IIPS 2005). Adults in rural areas were found to be more anaemic (7 percentage point difference for men and women) than those in urban areas. Education and economic status are both found to be positively correlated with levels of anaemia, so that among better educated men and women, and those from higher income backgrounds, the prevalence of anaemia is significantly lower. However, even among the most affluent sections of society, mild anaemia is prevalent, especially for girls. The primary reasons for iron deficiency anaemia are insufficient dietary intake of iron, poor iron absorption, repeated pregnancies and lactation among girls and women leading to increased iron requirements and poor iron reserves at birth (Anand et al. 2014).

A survey of 16 districts from 11 states of India done by Toteja et al. (2002) showed the overall prevalence of anaemia among adolescent girls to be as high as 90.1%. The prevalence of anaemia coexisted with deficiencies in other micronutrients like vitamin B-12 and folic acid. Thus, any intervention for adolescents and youth should not only target iron deficiency but deficiencies of other micronutrients also.

2.2.3.3 Zinc Deficiency

Zinc is one of the micronutrients which not only acts as a catalyst for enzymes, but its deficiency in the long run can result in permanent impairment in brain development and delayed sexual maturation. Zinc is essential for cellular metabolism, immune system functioning, cell division, protein and DNA synthesis (Food and Nutrition Board 2001). Zinc is also crucial for normal growth and development of the foetus and is essential during infancy, childhood and even into adolescence. Pregnant females and their young children are the most vulnerable to zinc deficiency, followed by older children and adolescents. Diets low in energy with poor bioavailability of dietary zinc are likely to be the primary cause of the high zinc deficiency among women (Herbst et al. 2014; Pathak et al. 2003; Agte et al. 2005), adolescents and youth (Kapil et al. 2011; Menon et al. 2011) in India. Although there are limited published studies on zinc deficiency among adolescents and young adults, they do indicate that the rates are fairly high.

2.2.3.4 Vitamin D and Calcium Deficiency

The requirement for vitamin D and calcium for skeletal development is far greater during adolescence than childhood or young adulthood. The adverse effects of calcium and vitamin D deficiency include rickets in childhood (skeletal disorder due to inadequate calcium, vitamin D or phosphate) and osteomalacia (condition that prevents bones from hardening and makes them more likely to break) or osteoporosis (condition where bones 'thin', also leading to higher likelihood of breaking) among adults. During adolescence, bone accrual takes place, and peak bone mass is achieved; therefore vitamin D is very crucial in this period. According to Rajeshwari et al. (2003), although India is a tropical country, there is poor exposure to sunshine due to social factors, which is compounded by low dietary calcium intake resulting in osteomalacia in adolescents. The findings on vitamin D deficiency indicate it is highly prevalent among adolescents in India and is more common in girls. Moreover, there are insufficient studies on young adult males and non-pregnant females. There is a need for effective and feasible vitamin D supplementation for prevention of hypovitaminosis D and for a prophylaxis for osteoporosis among adolescents and adults (Dhore and Wasnik 2013).

Besides iron, zinc and iodine, other minerals and trace elements that are essential in human nutrition are copper, magnesium and manganese. However, there is limited information on the occurrence of diet-related deficiencies in these minerals (Black 2001). There are also limited studies that have examined the prevalence of these mineral deficiencies among adolescents and youth.

2.2.4 Prevalence of Multiple Micronutrient Deficiencies

Due to limitations in the available data for adolescents and youth, it is difficult to estimate the prevalence of multiple MNDs among them. Muthayya et al. (2013) estimated the global hidden hunger indices for iron, vitamin A and zinc together and determined that 18 of the 20 countries with the highest burden of multiple MNDs are in Asia and Africa, including India. The research done on MNDs and multiple MNDs suggest that diets are often deficient in several micronutrients, including vitamins, and that supplementation with micronutrient mixtures is beneficial. In order to combat MNDs supplementation, fortification and food-based approaches like dietary diversification are generally used.

2.2.5 *Prevalence of Physical Activity*

In order to better tackle undernutrition and overweight and obesity, physical activity is an important component that needs to be studied further. The activity levels of an individual have an impact on the absorption of micronutrients. Extremely vigorous activity without sufficient intake can contribute to an individual becoming underweight, and inadequate physical activity with high caloric consumption can lead an individual to become overweight. In addition, physical activity can promote the absorption of micronutrients. Findings from a study done by Shah et al. (2013) in India suggest that children and adolescents who indulge in sedentary activities like watching TV, sitting in front of computers and playing video games are at higher risk of overweight and obesity. As is true in other countries, greater consumption of energy, fat, sweet and salty snacks and carbonated beverages, in addition to reducing the consumption of fruits and vegetables, has been found to be associated with excessive TV viewing and low physical activity (Rani and Sathiyasekaran 2013; Raj and Kumar 2010; Galhotra et al. 2008). Galhotra et al. (2008) has also posited that physical activity and time spent outdoors are notably low among adolescents in India because of the greater stress laid on academics at school. There are few interventions designed to increase physical activity among adolescents and even fewer among youth. Social, environmental and cultural factors play a large role in determining accessibility, availability and acceptability of physical activity among adolescent boys, and more so among girls.

2.2.6 *Gaps in Research and Data*

Numerous prevalence studies have highlighted the high percentages of adolescents who are underweight. However, there are fewer studies on the same among youth. More work is needed on the factors that lead to higher undernutrition among tribal populations. Additionally, as is evident from Table 2.3, there is a dearth of large-scale data on the prevalence of overweight and obesity among adolescents and, especially, youth. The data on differences between adolescents based on residence (urban vs. rural), sex and socioeconomic status are not fully understood. Still fewer studies have conclusively reported on differences in underweight and overweight based on caste, religion and parental education. Physical activity and its relationship with undernutrition and overweight and obesity remains a poorly studied area as well.

2.3 Government Policies and Programmes

2.3.1 National Nutrition Policy

The National Nutrition Policy (NNP) introduced in 1993 aimed to address the problem of undernutrition by utilising direct and indirect interventions to achieve short- and long-term nutritional goals. With a multisectoral approach, the NNP targets nutrition issues at various levels via direct and indirect interventions, as well as short- and long-term strategies. The NNP takes into consideration various problems like protein energy malnutrition, micronutrient deficiencies, low birth weight, overweight and undernutrition and strategies for natural calamities.

Vulnerable sections of the society, like children under 6 years of age, adolescent girls, pregnant and lactating women who are in dire need of nutrition supplementation are provided with food supplements as part of short-term direct interventions under NNP. Long-term indirect interventions like nutrition education, food fortification and growth monitoring are also provided as part of NNP and are not limited to only vulnerable sections of the society. The policy also highlights the following: land reforms; prevention of food adulteration; nutritional surveillance; health and family welfare; research; minimum wage administration; communication; community participation; equal remuneration for women; improvement of literacy, especially for women; and improving the status of women (Ministry of Women and Child Development 1993). Provision of health services like immunisation, antenatal care, postnatal care and basic health knowledge are also considered as indirect interventions.

Through long-term policy interventions, indirect factors like food security (ensuring production of 215 kg of food grain per person per year), improving dietary patterns and the purchasing power of rural and urban poor by public food distribution systems, and providing nutrition education were included. The NNP also included provisions for initiatives aimed at reaching out to adolescent girls, along with pregnant women by providing them proper nutrition to attain safe motherhood and to decrease the incidence of low birth weight babies. Provision of low-cost nutritious and fortified food and combating micronutrient deficiency in vulnerable groups were some of the short-term targets of the NNP.

The target populations for many of the programmes in India are children and married girls and women (primarily during pregnancy and while breastfeeding). Very few programmes and policies have taken adolescents in consideration, and none consider youth specifically. Some of the national food programmes are described below (Box 2.2).

2.3.2 The Integrated Child Development Scheme (ICDS)

Box 2.2 An Overview of the Integrated Child Development Scheme (ICDS)

The Integrated Child Development Scheme (ICDS) started on an experimental basis in only 33 blocks in 1975 but has grown rapidly and covers more than 90% of the blocks in the country today. Run by the Ministry of Women and Child Development (MWCD), ICDS is the largest outreach programme operational through Anganwadi centres (AWC).

Target population: Children (0–6 years), pregnant women and lactating mothers, women in reproductive age group (15–44 years) and adolescent girls

Objectives:

- Improve the nutritional and health status of children below the age of 6 years and that of pregnant and lactating mothers as well as of adolescent girls.
- Lay the foundations for proper psychological, physical and social development of the child.
- Reduce the incidence of mortality, morbidity, malnutrition and school dropout.
- Achieve effective coordination of policy and implementation among various departments to promote child development.

Enhance the capability of the mother to look after the normal health and nutritional needs of the child through proper health and nutrition education.

While several studies have looked at the effectiveness of the ICDS-run programmes, few have looked at specific components targeted at adolescents and youth. Findings on the effectiveness of the ICDS programmes suggest that the components on nutrition and health education are the most poorly implemented in comparison with the supplementation and food provision components. Chudasama et al. (2016) reported that 87% of the adolescent girls were availing ICDS services in Gujarat and there was high coverage of supplementary nutrition (SN) among pregnant mothers (84.6%), lactating mothers (84.6%) and adolescents (79.2%). Ready-to-eat food was provided to pregnant women (47.3%), lactating women (47.3%) and adolescent girls (46.4%), but the supply of take-home rations received was inadequate for all the beneficiaries of the Anganwadi centres (AWCs). Bredemkamp and Akin (2002) and Lokshin et al. (2005) found limited evidence based on differences between NFHS-1 and NFHS-2 data to support the positive impact of ICDS services and better child nutrition. According to Kandpal (2011), there is a need for better implementation of ICDS services, which might result in health and nutritional benefits for the beneficiaries. He reported that majority of the households used only the nutritional supplements, immunisation referral or day care facilities, which do not yield positive results. The Poverty Monitoring and Policy Support Unit (PMPSU) supported by DFID in Madhya Pradesh (MP) conducted an impact assessment of the Integrated Child Development Services (ICDS) in 2010. They found that only 28% of the adolescents were registered with the AWC for services under the adolescent scheme. A higher proportion of adolescents were registered in tribal blocks (34.7%) as compared to urban (29.1%) and rural blocks (20.9%). A majority of the registered adolescent girls (47.9%) reported distribution of supplementary nutrition by the AWC, followed by nutrition and health education (27.8%). Knowledge related to various schemes under ICDS was limited among the adolescent girls. In a rapid assessment of ICDS in Delhi, Sinha (2016), described the challenges, gaps and barriers faced by the chain of service providers. Although the supply of food through the supplementary nutrition programme was regular, the overall quality and nutrition content were not satisfactory. The nutrition composition of the diet was not satisfactory as there were limited vegetables in the food. Most of the times, the food was rich in carbohydrate and starch.

2.3.3 Midday Meal (MDM) Scheme

While majority of the beneficiaries of the MDM scheme are children, in many districts the MDM is provided to adolescents up to 10th grade. Although the need for school feeding programmes is the greatest in India, the overall coverage of school feeding programme is at 79% (World Food Program 2013). School feeding programmes contribute to a child's readiness to learn and ability to participate in his or her own educational process, and the benefits are particularly strong for girls (Box 2.3).

Box 2.3 Overview of the MDM Scheme
The Midday Meal (MDM) Scheme was started by the Ministry of Human Resource Development (HRD). It was launched as a centrally sponsored scheme on 15 August 1995 in order to enhance school enrolment, retention and attendance and to simultaneously improve the nutritional levels among children.

As of 2008, as part of the MDM scheme, every child in every government and government-aided primary and upper school (up to standard 8) is served a midday meal with a minimum content of 700 calories of energy and 20 grams of protein per day for a minimum of 200 days in a year.

MDM scheme is a direct approach to improve the nutritional status of children and adolescents in government and government-aided schools, (Mishra 2002; Dogra and Dogra 2003). In his study, Saxena (2003) claimed that the MDM programme has lowered the widespread incidence of malnutrition primarily among children of poor families and has increased their access to education. According to Saijhee (2003), almost all schools (95%) in Tamil Nadu reported that the midday meal programme has helped in increasing enrollment and retention of adolescent girls, but there was no significant improvement in their nutritional status. Sharma et al. (2010) reported significant improvement in the heights and weights of primary school students (aged 5–12 years) who were receiving wholesome midday meals in rural Uttar Pradesh. A comparison was made between the meal provided by a nongovernment organisation (NGO) and that provided by village panchayats. The authors reported that the midday meal provided by the NGO reduced the vitamin A and D deficiencies. The nutritional status of rural and urban school students (aged 5–15 years) receiving midday meals prepared by a Trust in schools of Bengaluru was studied by Shalini et al. (2014). They reported that the midday meal did have a positive impact on the nutritional status of children as the number and the degree of malnourishment would have been much greater in the absence of the scheme.

Bhargava et al. (2013) reported that the proportion of undernourished children among MDM beneficiaries of government schools were more (21.5%) in comparison with private schoolchildren who were beneficiaries (5.4%). The caloric content of school lunch was estimated to be 271 kcal in private school attendees and 375 kcal in MDM beneficiaries. The calorie content of diets was more in MDM beneficiaries due to cereal and pulse combination, but it lacked fruits and vegetables. It was found that higher numbers of older children beyond class VIII tend to skip lunch in government schools in comparison with those in private schools. Bhargava et al. (2013) highlighted the need to focus on the quality of lunch in schools and detailed nutritional surveys for acquiring richer research data.

In a Cochrane review, Kristjansson et al. (2007) found that school feeding programmes significantly improved the school attendance levels and the growth and cognitive performance of disadvantaged children globally. Patel et al. (2016) evaluated the effect of the MDM programme on the nutritional status of adolescents (10–14 years) and compared them with a healthy comparison group of adolescents from private schools. It was found that the percentage of wasting (17% boys and 18% girls) and stunting (24% boys and 19% girls) was significantly higher in adolescents receiving the MDM. It was found that the MDM receiving adolescents were vulnerable to energy, protein as well as micronutrient deficiencies.

The MDM scheme has helped in improving the attendance of children and adolescents in schools, in imparting education and assuring nutrition to the backward sections of the society; however, a comprehensive and elaborate mechanism for monitoring and supervision of the MDM scheme is essential for complete eradication of malnutrition. Apart from this, emphasis must be given for facilitating safe drinking water, hygiene and sanitation facilities within the school. Intervention programmes to fill the gaps between the approval and coverage of schools are needed (Maneesh 2015). According to Nambiar et al. (2012a, b), the MDM programme has shown partial success, and improvement is required for better infrastructure and facilities in schools along with training of the MDM staff. The nutritional quality and quantity of the meal need to be improved as research studies have shown very high prevalence of micronutrient deficiencies, unhygienic cooking conditions and high prevalence of infections (Nambiar and Desai 2013; Nambiar et al. 2012a, b; Nambiar and Desai 2012) (Box 2.4).

Box 2.4 An Overview of the PDS

The Public Distribution System (PDS) was started by the Ministry of Consumer Affairs, Food and Civil Supplies with the aim of providing food security to Indians. PDS is a targeted scheme that provides specified quantities of selected commodities (wheat, rice, sugar and kerosene) at subsidised prices through a network of fair price shops to households who are below the poverty line.

Objectives

1. To provide food grains and other essential items to vulnerable sections of the society at reasonable (subsidised) prices
2. To put an indirect check on the open market prices of various items
3. To attempt socialisation in the matter of distribution of essential commodities

2.3.4 Public Distribution System

According to a Performance Evaluation by the planning commission (PEO 2005), PDS has not been effective in ensuring food security to the needy. Ray and Ray (2011) highlighted several problems with the targeted PDS (TPDS) such as large-scale exclusion of genuinely needy people from the PDS, poor functioning of delivery system and no price stabilisation through transfer of cereals from surplus to deficit regions of the country. Due to extensive leakages, commodities do not reach the people in need. Evaluation studies on the link between PDS and nutrient intake have contrasting results. Kochar (2005) found that greater income transfer through the PDS did not lead to greater calorie consumption for the targeted households. Kaushal and Muchomba (2013) found no significant relationship between higher nutritional intake and PDS participation, but Krishnamurthy et al. (2014) reported higher nutrient intake and diet quality among the beneficiaries in Chhattisgarh. Kaushal and Muchomba (2013) also evaluated the impact of the transition from universal to a targeted PDS on nutritional intake using nationally representative data for the period 1993–1994 and 2009–2010 but did not find any effect of the greater consumer subsidy from PDS on total calorie intake. In general, studies on the effectiveness of PDS have examined it from a household perspective, and the impact on individual food security has not been assessed. Thus, there are no studies that have looked at food security outcomes for adolescents or youth separately as a direct outcome of the PDS.

Although PDS has failed in certain sections, it is assumed to play a major role by ensuring access to certain minimum quantities of grains and other commodities throughout the country and in all seasons at uniform prices. For effective implementation of PDS, there is a need to recognise differences in needs and problems across states so that the delivery system can be improved for effective implementation and to reduce leakages.

2.3.5 Rashtriya Kishor Swasthya Karyakram (RKSK): National Adolescent Health Programme

The vision of RKSK is to improve their health by enabling adolescents to realise their full potential by making informed and responsible decisions. Adolescent participation and leadership have been prioritised by RKSK along with gender equity in partnership with other sectors and stakeholders. The MOHFW has collaborated with UNFPA for effective implementation of this programme. A National Adolescent Health Strategy was originally devised and, then, translated into the RKSK programme. This programme works intersectorally with other ministries and with the state governments. The emphasis of the RKSK programme is based on seven 'Cs,' i.e. communities, coverage, content, communication, counselling, clinics and convergence. The strength of the programme lies in its focus on health promotion. RKSK has introduced community-based interventions through peer educators, to educate and inform the adolescents about nutrition, sexual and reproductive health, mental health, substance misuse and injuries (Box 2.5).

Box 2.5 An Overview of the RKSK Programme
The MOHFW launched a health programme specially targeting adolescents in the age group of 10–19 years in January 2014. The programme is supposed to target the nutritional needs, reproductive health, substance abuse, violence (including gender-based violence), non-communicable diseases and mental health of the adolescents. RKSK reaches out to both young males and females, married and unmarried, in and out of school from rural and urban parts of India.

The package of services provided under the RKSK is divided into community- and facility-based interventions. Services which come under community-based interventions are Peer Education (PE), Quarterly Adolescent Health Day (AHD), Weekly Iron and Folic Acid Supplementation Programme (WIFS) and Menstrual Hygiene Scheme (MHS). Under community-based interventions, four trained peer educators (PEs) are selected to provide commodities and to support and impart information and education to the adolescents living in the community. The services of the Adolescent Friendly Health Clinics (AFHC) are provided under facility-based interventions.

As the RKSK is a relatively new programme, there are no published studies that have examined the effectiveness, reach or efficacy of this programme. In addition, the rollout of various components of the programme varies across the states and, even, across districts. Thus, there is a need for better monitoring and information about this programme.

2.4 Programmes to Address Micronutrient Deficiencies

2.4.1 Iron Deficiency/Anaemia

The National Anemia Control Programme (NACP) began in 1991. Since then, the programme has been changed to the Weekly Iron and Folic Acid Supplementation (WIFS) programme, which has been subsumed under the National Rural Health Mission (NRHM) and subsequently under RKSK in some parts of the country. There are programmatic and organisational issues that have hampered the success of the anaemia control programme (Anand et al. 2014) (Box 2.6).

Box 2.6 An Overview of the National Anemia Control Programmes in India

The National Nutritional Anaemia Control Programme (NNACP) was launched in 1991 by Ministry of Health and Family Welfare, GOI with the following objectives:

- To assess the baseline prevalence of nutritional anaemia in mothers and young children through estimation of haemoglobin (Hb) levels
- To put the mothers and children with low Hb levels (less than 10 g and less than 8 g respectively) on anti-anaemia treatment
- To put the mother with Hb level more than 10 g/dl and children with Hb more than 8 g/dl on the prophylaxis programme
- To monitor continuously the quality of the tablets, distribution and consumption of the supplements
- To assess periodically the Hb levels of the beneficiaries
- To motivate the mothers to consume the tablets (and to give to their children also) through relevant nutrition education

(continued)

Box 2.6 (continued)

The Weekly Iron and Folic Acid Supplementation (WIFS) programme aims to reduce the prevalence and severity of anaemia in the adolescent population (10–19 years), with high priority given to both school-going and non-school-going adolescent girls in government or municipal schools (in the 6th to 12th standards) in both urban and rural areas.

In the original programme, the target population included married, pregnant and non-pregnant adolescent girls. Under the NHM, WIFS is administered for 52 weeks of the year. The WIFS programme provides information on how to improve diets, increase iron intake in food as well as iron absorption along with counselling and support to adolescent girls (WIFS, National Health Mission, MOHFW, GOI).

This has been taken over by the Rashtriya Kishor Swasthya Karyakram which provides iron supplements to adolescent boys in schools also. However, this has not been implemented all over the country.

2.4.2 *Iodine Deficiency*

Deficiency of iodine affects the entire life course from infancy to adulthood (Zimmermann 2009). Iodine deficiency impacts the functioning of the thyroid gland and leads to goitre (enlargement of the thyroid gland) and other complications. Pregnant females and infants (<24 months of age) are the population groups at highest risk of iodine deficiency, followed by adolescents and young adults. Thirty percent of the world's school-aged children have insufficient iodine intake (Pfeiffer et al. 2007). In order to prevent iodine deficiency, universal salt iodisation is the most practical and effective approach, not only in India, but all over the world. Correcting iodine deficiency does have some health risks for certain populations in terms of thyroid function and should be considered within the context of each country separately (Zimmermann et al. 2008). At present, the household-level iodised salt coverage in India is 91%, although 71% of the households actually consume adequately iodised salt (Pandav et al. 2013). There are few studies that examine intro-household consumption of iodine (Box 2.7).

Box 2.7 Overview of the National Iodine Deficiency Programme in India
The National Iodine Deficiency Disorder Control Programme was introduced in 1992, to reduce the prevalence of iodine deficiency disorders below 10% in the entire country by 2012. The focus of NIDDCP was on production, demand and supply of iodised salt for universal consumption by the entire country. The key problem of NIDDCP was to reach the vulnerable populations.

(continued)

Box 2.7 (continued)

The following are the components of NIDDCP policy and programme:

- Undertake periodic surveys to assess the magnitude of the problem.
- Ensure supply of iodised salt in place of common salt to the entire population for edible purposes.
- Organise health education and publicity to promote consumption of iodised salt.
- Establish laboratory monitoring of iodised salt and urinary iodine.
- Resurvey after 5 years to assess the extent of iodine deficiency disorders and the impact of iodised salt.

2.4.3 Other Micronutrients

There are no national or state programmes for supplementation to prevent or treat VAD among adolescents or youth. Since 2006, the vitamin A prophylaxis programme offered by the Ministry of Health and Family Welfare (MoHFW) includes the provision of six monthly administrations of vitamin A syrup to children between the ages of 6 months and 5 years.

Zinc is given to infants and children when treated for diarrhoea, but there is no programme specifically targeting zinc supplements among adolescents. There are no programmes that offer vitamin D or calcium supplementation to adolescents or young adults. There are no national or state programmes that offer supplementation for multiple MNDs for adolescents or youth. Fortified food is provided for underweight children and pregnant girls and women via the food supplementation programmes mentioned above. There is an increase in the number of schemes planned for young people, but access to them is still poor due to the prevailing inequitable gender and social norms (Sivagurunathan et al. 2015). There is an urgent need to improve the accessibility of these schemes for adolescents, as well as improve the utilisation patterns in order to improve their nutritional status and well-being. Yet more crucial is the necessity to make young people aware of these schemes enhancing their reach to the available opportunities, provisions, information and skills.

2.4.4 Gaps in Research and Data

As is apparent from the descriptions earlier, there is some data on several micronutrient deficiencies among adolescents and youth. However, there are no micronutrient supplementation programmes for adolescents or youth. The biggest exception to this is iron deficiency, for which multiple programmes have been launched targeting adolescent girls and now, boys as well. However, research suggests that the concomitant activities to improve awareness about iron deficiency have not been done, which has led to poorer uptake of the iron supplements and poorer compliance. This is aside from the logistical and administrative issues with procurement and distribution of iron tablets, which has hampered the successful implementation and performance of the iron supplementation programmes. Much work needs to be done on improving the accessibility of the programme and reducing bottlenecks within the system. Within the PDS and certain schemes, there is an attempt to provide fortified food to the public, but the effectiveness of these efforts and the implementation across the country have not been well-studied. In addition, there are some researchers who question the sustainability and effectiveness of a supplementation model. They believe that the government needs to promote agriculture that provides the micronutrients via food intake in addition to providing fortified food via PDS. Most importantly, there is a dearth of research on the short-term and long-term implications of micronutrient deficiencies among adolescents and youth.

2.5 Vulnerable Adolescents and Youth

Research on the nutritional status and needs of adolescents and youth with special needs in India, such as those living with tuberculosis (TB), human immunodeficiency virus (HIV) and/or acquired immunodeficiency syndrome (AIDS), those with physical disabilities, those diagnosed with mental illnesses and individuals suffering from cancer and those living in institutions, is inadequate. There is a need to address these vulnerable groups, so that the neglect they experience in other ways is not compounded by neglect in the area of nutrition.

HIV in children and adolescents is often accompanied by co-morbid conditions such as anaemia, malnutrition and opportunistic infections. The increased energy demands make HIV patients more vulnerable to deficiencies of micronutrients such as iron and vitamins A and B complex. Anaemia is very common in children and adolescents with HIV infection and is an independent marker for increased disease progression and death in children, adolescents and adults (Shet et al. 2009; Shah et al. 2005). Undernutrition is also common among those who are HIV positive and is associated with poorer outcomes, and an improvement in nutritional status leads to better clinical outcomes (Semba 2003). With proper nutrition, disease progression is reported to be delayed, which could postpone the need for antiretroviral therapy (ART) and preserve long-term therapeutic options for the patient (Fawzi et al. 2004). Studies specifically targeting adolescents and youth are very scarce in India. The research done globally indicates a need for proper nutrition intervention among HIV-infected adolescents and youth in India.

Not much research on the incidence of TB in adolescents in India has been done, although it has been reported that the risk of acquiring TB disease after TB infection is higher in adolescents compared to adults (Global TB Report 2015). According to Padmapriyadarsini et al. (2016), nutrition and tuberculosis are interrelated. Undernutrition can increase the risk of TB, which in turn can lead to malnutrition. In studies with adults (Bhargava et al. 2013), stunting and wasting are commonly seen at the time of diagnosis, and this persists until the end of treatment.

As there is little data on TB among adolescents, there is a need to examine their nutrition needs and provide support for greater improvement at the time of treatment. Nutrition has an important role to play in both the prevention and control of TB. The bidirectional relationship between TB and nutrition should be studied further and tackled in the national programme, especially for populations that are highly vulnerable.

Type 2 diabetes mellitus (T2DM) is linked to behavioural, nutritional and environmental factors and has emerged as the leading cause of chronic illness, disability and death even in developing countries like India. The incidence of T2DM in children and adolescents in India has increased markedly, and it accounts for one third of all the new cases of diabetes diagnosed in adolescents (Vikram et al. 2006). In their study, Bhatia (2004) reported 12% of cases of T2DM among adolescents below 18 years. The dietary requirements of T2DM among adolescents and youth vary from those of adults as they are growing. In addition, being a juvenile population, the understanding of the chronicity of the disease and the requirements of management are harder to explain and understand. There is little research on the management of the disease among adolescents and on factors that lead to better dietary practices in Indian young adult populations.

Children with mental illnesses are at high risk of developing undernutrition and micronutrient deficiencies, which can result in growth retardation and other complications later in life. A study conducted by Mathur et al. (2007) among 7–18-year-olds found that more children with a diagnosis of intellectual disability were underweight than children without a diagnosis and the prevalence of overweight was more in those children who were not intellectually disabled. It was observed that children with intellectual disability had difficulty in chewing and swallowing and they had a tendency to spit out and vomit food. The diets of children with intellectual disability were deficient in iron and riboflavin and that of non-diagnosed children in iron only. Even the extent of disability was associated with self-feeding practices. Seena and Ramadas (2002) found that children with 'Down's syndrome' were shorter than normal children. Younger children weighed less and had deficient calorie intake, whereas older children (10–16 years) weighed more and had surplus calorie intake than children without Down's syndrome. There was insufficient intake of protein and vitamins A, C and B complex and excessive intake of fat among younger and older children. Aggarwal et al. (2015) reported that the micronutrient deficiency and stunting levels of children with cerebral palsy were much higher in developing countries than in developed countries. Inadequate dietary intake, feeding problems, socioeconomic status, and disease severity were some of the causative factors highlighted by the authors.

Adolescents living in orphanages or institutes are more at risk of being undernourished or having micronutrient deficiencies than an adolescent living at home (Deininger et al. 2003). A study done by UNICEF indicated that orphans are more likely to have growth and development deficiencies, remain nutritionally undernourished and are less likely to be enrolled in school than children living with both parents (Deininger et al. 2003). Orphans are more vulnerable because of poor nutrition and incomplete access to health services. Thus, they are at increased risk of starvation, illness and death. In one study, it was found that the menu provided at orphanages was dense in calories but deficient in micronutrients due to lack of proteins, green leafy vegetables and fruits (Lone and Ganesan 2016).

In addition to orphanages, adolescents and youth in institutional setups including halfway homes, juvenile detention centres and jails are underserved as a result of being institutionalised. Their poor nutritional status increases their vulnerability to increased morbidity and poorer socioeconomic status even after they leave the institutional setup. There is no published research done on the nutrition status or deficiencies of adolescents and youth who are in institutions in India. This is a sizeable research gap and serves to compound the lack of importance given to this group of adolescents.

2.6 Factors Affecting Food Intake

In their multistate study in Rural India, NNMB (2012) assessed the diet of adolescents and young adults. The average daily intake of food and nutrients was assessed among 10–17-year-olds and showed that on average, the intake of cereals and millets and pulses was lower than the Recommended Dietary Allowances (RDA) for Indians as suggested by the Indian Council of Medical Research (ICMR) expert committee (2010). An increasing trend was noted in the consumption of fruits, green leafy vegetables, fats and oils over the years. Time trends of food consumption among adolescents and young adults showed a substantial reduction in intake of cereals, roots and tubers, milk and milk products, sugar and jaggery and certain vegetables over the last four decades. These findings need further elucidation to understand the structural, familial, societal and individual factors that lead to changes in food choices and consumption among adolescents and youth. In addition, there are few studies that look at food and nutrition security among adolescents and even fewer look at it among young adults.

Many factors determine food choice and intake among adolescents and youth, like socioeconomic status, culture, region, sex and age. In addition, adolescents' choice of foods is influenced by the media, family, peers and knowledge. Recent studies have indicated that faulty eating behaviour and dietary factors, along with lack of physical activity can not only result in obesity among young adults but can also lead to insulin resistance syndrome, hypertension, dyslipidemia, hypertriglyceridemia and poor micronutrient status (Nawab et al. 2014; Jagadesan et al. 2014; Kotian et al. 2010; Stigler 2011; Gupta et al. 2011).

The socioeconomic status (SES) of an individual plays a crucial role in the food decision-making, buying practices and consumption. Studies have shown a negative relationship between SES and undernutrition. Higher levels of undernutrition have been associated with lower SES. Similar findings were observed in studies done by Sidhu et al. (2005), Laxmaiah et al. (2007), Aggarwal et al. (2008) and Gupta et al. (2011). Mean intake of energy, protein, fat, calcium, vitamin D and milk/milk products was significantly higher in upper socioeconomic strata than lower strata girls. Conversely, carbohydrate, fibre, phytate and cereal intakes were higher in lower socioeconomic groups rather than upper socioeconomic strata girls, as the sources of these foods are cheaper and easily accessible.

Mondala et al. (2012) conducted a study with children and adolescents (6–16 years) and found gender discrimination against the females resulting in higher rates of undernutrition. They found that girls were rated undernourished on the basis of predictors like father's occupational status, per capita income, number of siblings and number of rooms, but this was not the case among the boys. Females were found to be consuming less nutrient rich diets than males and were twice as likely to suffer from micronutrient deficiencies revealing sizeable gender inequalities (IIPS 2007; Arnold et al. 2009). Substantial research points to a gender gap in undernutrition levels as well as in micronutrient deficiencies. These cannot be explained by biological and physiological differences. Thus, social, cultural and economic factors influence household food allocation and lead to poorer food consumption among girls. There is insufficient research on how this continues into young adulthood, and no programme addresses this causative factor contributing to undernutrition among girls.

Chugh and Puri (2001) conducted a study to compare eating and weight concerns among underweight, normal-weight and overweight adolescent girls (16–18 years) in New Delhi. Even normal weight and underweight girls reported concerns about excess weight. The level of satisfaction with body size decreased with increase in weight. A higher number of obese (76.6%) compared with normal-weight (38%), and underweight (14%) girls reported that they engaged in dieting. These adolescent girls were found to be missing meals, snacking and eating out. Johnson et al. (2015) assessed the nutritional status and body image perception of adolescents in rural south India. It was found that 63% of the participants had normal BMI for age, 32% were undernourished and 5% were overweight and obese. However, more than half (53%) of them wished they were thinner and 52% taller. Seventy-nine percent of the participants were found to have body image dissatisfaction. Majority of undernourished adolescents (70.3%) perceived themselves to be normal, while 66.7% of overweight adolescents perceived themselves to be normal. Negative body image perception and body image dissatisfaction is very common in adolescence and frequently leads to unhealthy eating habits like skipping meals, which in turn can exacerbate poor nutrition status and lead to eating disorders like bulimia and anorexia. There are no large-scale published studies that examine body image dissatisfaction among adolescent boys and youth; however, in urban areas, there is a focus on increasing muscularity, which is associated with unhealthy eating habits and use of steroids.

2.7 Knowledge, Awareness and Media Influences

In addition to food supplementation, nutrition education is used as a way of promoting lifelong healthy eating practices among children and adolescents. According to Ambre and Sengupta (2015), the occurrence of nutritional problems like anaemia, protein energy malnutrition (PEM) and rickets develops due to lack of knowledge and awareness which leads to faulty eating practices. They conducted a nutrition education programme (NEP) among adolescent girls and found a significant improvement in nutritional knowledge of the adolescent girls after exposure to the programme. In a study done by Tharkar and Viswanathan (2009) among adolescents, the levels of knowledge and awareness about healthy lifestyles were poor and did not show a significant association with overweight or obesity. Mean knowledge scores among younger adolescents and girls in upper socioeconomic strata were better in comparison to respondents from lower-income backgrounds.

Rani et al. (2013) assessed the knowledge and practices of high school students with respect to healthy diets before and after a nutrition education programme in Chennai, India. Post-nutrition education programme, dietary knowledge significantly improved from 37% to 67%, and attitude towards healthy diet increased from 18% to 40%. The intake of soft drinks and fast-food consumption also halved after the intervention suggesting that the provision of nutrition information can impact diet. Rao et al. (2007a, b) assessed the dietary habits and nutrition knowledge levels of adolescent girls and studied the efficacy of two different nutrition education tools in improving their nutrition knowledge in Hyderabad, India. Food frequency questionnaire data revealed more consumption of aerated drinks, bakery items and fast foods and less consumption of millets irrespective of their socioeconomic conditions. Consumption of vegetables, green leafy vegetables and fruits was moderate. Significant improvement in the nutrition-related knowledge was observed among the experimental group after the education intervention (in two forms – via traditional media and via audio-visual CDs) as compared to the baseline data. In a school-based programme conducted by Shah et al. (2010), children and adolescents (8–18 years) were educated about health, nutrition, physical activity, non-communicable diseases and healthy cooking practices in three cities of North India. Baseline data revealed low nutrition knowledge scores in government (75–94%) and private (48–78%) schools.

An impact evaluation done by the NNMB (2012) showed that despite the implementation of various national nutrition programmes at the community level, only 14% of the adolescent population had been exposed to nutrition education due to poor implementation of IEC. The review of literature revealed major gaps in health- and nutrition-related knowledge and behaviour of children and adolescents.

The nutrition and media literacy report (2009) revealed that children are exposed to around 7600 food commercials a year on television. Between 35% and 45% of the commercials on television are for food advertisements. Commercials increase preference for advertised foods and increase children's requests to parents for those foods. Out of the total food advertisements that are shown during television programmes, healthy food advertisements (e.g. milk and milk products, fortified wheat flour and biscuits, cereal based products/cornflakes) constitute only 4%, while majority of the advertised products are high in fats and calories. Maheshwar and Vijayapushpam (2014) analysed food advertisements on children's channels and found that 43% of foods advertisements were of chocolates and sweets, followed by fast food (11.6%), health/energy drinks (10.5%) and biscuits (10%). Ghimire and Rao (2013) and Gupta et al. (2017) also observed that majority of food advertising content watched by young adolescents on television is related to calorie dense and micronutrient-deficient foods and beverages.

2.8 Recommendations

Based on the review, it can be inferred that adolescents and youth require further nutrition interventions, especially in the form of better designed IEC or education activities, besides proper health care, to improve their health and nutrition status. As is apparent from the data presented in this review, there is adequate epidemiological evidence on the nutrition status of adolescents. However, there are certain vulnerable sections of adolescents whose nutrition status is inadequately studied. There is a need to examine youth as a separate demographic group. Most importantly, there are a dearth of programmes that target micronutrient deficiencies among adolescents and youth and factors affecting food intake are poorly understood. In addition, the implementation of newer programmes for adolescents that include nutrition components points to the fact that the government is cognisant of the necessity of focusing on this segment of the population. The relative lack of attention to designing programmes for young adults is more worrisome.

2.8.1 Policy Level

(1) The National Nutrition Policy (NNP) was formulated in 1993 and covered nutrition sensitive and specific interventions through the life course, highlighting the nutritional needs for adolescents and youth on paper. However, this was not translated into programmes that led to effective results. The NNP needs to be updated to reflect the nutrition transition (increase in prevalence of overweight and obesity), and there needs to be special focus on adolescents and young adult boys.

(2) The focal point of all existing programmes and policies are directed towards the delivery of supplementary nutrition, but emphasis must be given for facilitating safe drinking water, hygiene and sanitation facilities. Indirect interventions such as WASH, education, food security and agriculture should also be included within the policy frameworks for long-term sustenance of the short-term strategies. Food security among adolescents and youth should be examined separately.

(3) *The Dietary Guidelines for Indians* (National Institute of Nutrition 2011) do not match the WHO guidelines of dietary intake of fruits and vegetables for adolescents (400 g) and other country guidelines of five servings a day. These need to be updated and communicated to the public.

(4) As part of the process of designing policies on nutrition, a health impact assessment would be helpful in making a stronger case for policies and programmes that specifically target adolescent and youth nutrition. This would establish the short-term and long-term benefits of working in this area and lead to overall development in the country.

2.8.2 Programmatic

(1) There is a need to develop a state- and/or national-level database regarding uptake of programmes among adolescents and their health and nutrition status. Such a large-scale database will help in developing an integrated approach to address the nutritional problems of adolescents and youth.
(2) An inter-sectoral approach is an important first step in devising any programmes for adolescents and youth. Strategies need to be devised to include and integrate nutrition into existing programmes that target this segment of the population. There is a dire need for inclusive strategies and specific policies targeting adolescents and youth at the national level to define priorities and to integrate nutrition concerns into existing programmes reaching adolescents and youth. This can include school-based interventions. Regular nutritional screening, micronutrient supplementation intervention and nutrition education can be successfully implemented in schools and colleges. It is important to note that since there are large numbers of adolescents and youth who are not in school, programmes have to cater to the needs of those who are out of school as well.
(3) In order to better understand the situation, adolescents and youth should be actively involved in the design, planning, implementation and evaluation of programmes that aim to improve their health and nutritional status, which will also increase their ownership.
(4) The exploration of best practices would be an insightful exercise in order to improve programmes. In some cases, states and districts within states have met with partial success with innovative strategies, and it is worthy of investigation to see how these can be mainstreamed and implemented on a large scale. The fact that there is wide interstate variation in nutrition status and also in uptake of programmes suggests that governance and political will can have an impact on the effectiveness of the programmes.
(5) In addition to including components related to food safety within the national policy, there should be greater incorporation of information and education about safe and sanitary practices for water and food storage into national programmes for adolescents and youth.
(6) Physical activity remains relatively neglected in the discourses on nutrition among adolescents and youth. With increasing rates of overweight and obesity along with increases in the risk for diabetes and cardiovascular conditions, it is imperative that nutrition programmes include components on physical activity for adolescents and youth, especially in urban areas.

2.8.3 Community and Media-based approaches

(1) Dietary guidelines formulated by the NIN have not been disseminated enough to the public or to public health professionals. There are a variety of modalities by which this can be done including using community and media-based approaches.
(2) The media has the power to influence the dietary intake and eating behaviour of the population, especially adolescents and youth. Multimedia approaches can be used to develop an educational programme discussing the importance of healthy eating habits, balanced diet and physical activity as well as the promotion of fortified foods that could be imparted through food advertisements, brochures, songs, slogans, videos, leaflets and pamphlets.
(3) Social marketing of nutritious foods can also be done to inform, educate and motivate adolescents and youth about different food groups, dietary diversity, healthy lifestyle and eating behaviour.
(4) As is apparent from studies done on food choice and intake, adolescents and youth often make food choices that may not be healthy. The impact of advertising cannot be understated in influencing their choices. Teaching them to be media savvy, read labels and create greater awareness about the value of food labels is an important exercise.
(5) Community-level interventions that have improved food intake, increased physical activity and contributed to better growth indicators need to be examined critically with a view to understanding the processes and mechanisms that are effective in engaging adolescents and youth and bringing about positive change.

References

Agarwal, K. N., Gomber, S., Bisht, H., & Som, M. (2003). Anemia prophylaxis in adolescent school girls by weekly or daily iron-folate supplementation. *Indian Pediatrics, 40(4)*, 296–301.

Aggarwal, T., Bhatia, R. C., Singh, D., & Sobti, P. C. (2008). Prevalence of obesity and overweight in affluent adolescents from Ludhiana, Punjab. *Indian Pediatrics, 45*, 500–502.

Aggarwal, S., Chadha, R., & Pathak, R. (2015). Nutritional status and growth in children with cerebral palsy: A review. *International Journal of Medicine Science & Public Health, 5*, 737–744.

Agte, V., Chiplonkar, S., & Tarwadi, K. (2005). Factors influencing zinc status of apparently healthy Indians. *Journal of the American College of Nutrition, 24*, 334–341.

Ambre, S. P., & Sengupta, R. (2015). Effect of nutrition education program on dietary eating patterns of adolescent girls (16-19 years). *International Journal of Pure Applied Biosciences, 3(2)*, 427–431.

Anand, P., Rahi, M., Sharma, P., & Ingle, K. (2014). Issues in prevention of iron deficiency in anemia in India. *Nutrition, 30*(7–8), 764–770.

Arnold, F., Parasuraman, S., Arokiasamy, P., & Kothari, M. (2009). *Nutrition in India*. National Family Health Survey (NFHS-3), India, 2005-06, Mumbai/Calverton, MD: International Institute for Population Sciences and ICF Macro.

Balgir, R. S., Kerketta, A. S., Murmu, B., & Dash, B. P. (2002). Clinical assessment of health and nutritional status of Gond children in Kalahandi district of Orissa. *Indian Journal of Nutrition & Diet, 39*, 31–37.

Banerji, M. A., Faridi, N., Atluri, R., Chaiken, R. L., & Lebovitz, H. E. (1999). Body composition, visceral fat, leptin and insulin resistance in Asian Indian men. *Journal of Clinical Endocrinology & Metabolism, 84*, 137–144.

Banik, S. D. (2009). Health and nutritional status of three adult male populations of Eastern India: An anthropometric appraisal. *Italian Journal of Public Health, 6*, 294–302.

Bansal, P. G., Toteja, G. S., Bhatia, N., Vikram, N. K., Siddhu, A., Garg, A. K., & Roy, A. K. (2016). Deficiencies of serum ferritin and vitamin B12, but not folate, are common in adolescent girls residing in a slum in Delhi. *International Journal for Vitamin and Nutrition Research, 85*, 14–22. https://doi.org/10.1024/0300-9831/a000219.

Bhambhani, G. D., Bhambhani, R. G., & Thakor, N. C. (2015). Health profile of adolescents of Bhavnagar district, Gujarat, India: A cross sectional study. *International Journal of Respiratory Medicine Sciences, 3*, 3372–3376.

Bharati, D. R., Deshmukh, P. R., & Garg, B. S. (2008). Correlates of overweight & obesity among school going children of Wardha city, Central India. *Indian Journal of Medical Research, 127(6)*, 539–543.

Bhardwaj, S., Misra, A., Khurana, L., Gulati, S., Shah, P., & Vikram, N. K. (2008). Childhood obesity in Asian Indians: A burgeoning cause of insulin resistance, diabetes and sub-clinical inflammation. *Asia Pacific Journal of Clinical Nutrition, 17(S1)*, 172–175.

Bhargava, A., Chatterjee, M., Jain, Y., Chatterjee, B., Kataria, A., et al. (2013). Nutritional status of adult patients with pulmonary tuberculosis in Rural Central India and its association with mortality. *PLOS ONE, 8(10)*, e77979. https://doi.org/10.1371/journal.pone.0077979.

Bhatia, V. (2004). IAP National task force for childhood prevention of adult diseases. Insulin resistance and type 2 diabetes mellitus in childhood. *Indian Pediatrics, 41*, 443–457.

Black, R. E. (2001). Micronutrients in pregnancy. *British Journal of Nutrition, 85*(Suppl. 2), S193–S197.

Brendemkamp, C., & Akin, J. S. (2002). *India's integrated child development services scheme: Meeting health and nutritional needs of children, adolescent girls and women*. Washington, DC: World Bank.

Chaitali, G., Mangala, S., Hemalatha, A. J., Pradeep, C., & Subrahmanyam, G. (2014). Childhood and adolescent overweight and obesity – A public health challenge in India. *International Journal of Scientific Studies, 2(4)*, 17–19.

Chakrabarty, S., & Bharati, P. (2010). Nutritional status among the Shabar tribal children living in urban, rural and forest habitats of Orissa, India. *Italian Journal of Public Health, Volume, 7(3)*, 303–310.

Chaudhary, C., Pathak, R., Ahluwalia, S. K., Goel, R. K. D., & Devgan, S. (2013). Iodine deficiency disorder in children aged 6-12 years of Ambala, Haryana. *Indian Pediatrics, 50(6)*, 587–589.

Chhatwal, J., Verma, M., & Riar, S. K. (2004). Obesity among pre-adolescent and adolescents of a developing country (India). *Asia Pacific Journal of Clinical Nutrition, 3*, 231–235.

Chudasama, R. K., Patel, U. V., Kadri, A. M., Mitra, A., Thakkar, D., & Oza, J. (2016). Evaluation of integrated child development services program in Gujarat, India for the years 2012 to 2015. *Indian Journal of Public Health, 60(2)*, 124–130. https://doi.org/10.4103/0019-557X.184544.

Chugh, R., & Puri, S. (2001). Affluent adolescent girls of Delhi: Eating and weight concerns. *British Journal of Nutrition, 86*, 535–542.

Consortium for Media Literacy. (2009). *Nutrition and media literacy report*. http://www.medialit.org/sites/default/files/connections/media%20literacy%20and%20nutrition.pdf. Accessed on 18th September, 2016.

Deininger, K., Garcia, M., & Subbarao, K. (2003). AIDS-induced orphanhood as a systemic shock: Magnitude, impact, and program interventions in Africa. *World Development., 31*, 1201–1220.

Deshmukh, P. R., Gupta, S. S., Bharambe, M. S., Dongre, A. R., Maliye, C., Kaur, S., et al. (2006). Nutritional status of adolescents in rural Wardha. *Indian Journal of Pediatrics, 73*, 139–141.

Dhore, R., & Wasnik, V. (2013). Vitamin D status of apparently healthy early adolescents in Amravati City of Maharashtra, India. *International Journal of Collaborative Research on Internal Medicine & Public Health, 5*(9), 608–618.

Dogra, M., & Dogra, B. (2003). *Reforming the mid-day meal programme*. www.righttofood.com. Accessed on 19th August, 2016.

Fawzi, W. W., Msamanga, G. I., Spiegelman, D., Wei, R., Kapiga, S., Villamor, E., Mwakagile, D., Mugusi, F., Hertzmark, E., Essex, M., & Hunter, D. J. (2004). A randomized trial of multivitamin supplements and HIV disease progression and mortality. *New England Journal of Medicine, 351*(*1*), 23–32.

Food and Nutrition Board. (2001). *Dietary reference intakes for Vitamin A, Vitamin K, Arsenic, Boron, Chromium, Copper, Iodine, Iron, Manganese, Molybdenum, Nickel, Silicon, Vanadium, and Zinc*. Washington DC: National Academy Press.

Galhotra, A., Abrol, A., Agarwal, N., Goel, N. K., & Gupta, S. (2008). Lifestyle related risk factors for cardiovascular diseases in Indian adolescents. *The Internet Journal of Health, 9*(2), 1–5. http://ispub.com/IJH/9/2/4263.

Garg, M. K., Tandon, N., Marwaha, R. K., Menon, A. S., & Mahalle, N. (2013). The relationship between serum 25-hydroxy vitamin D, parathormone and bone mineral density in Indian population. *Clinical Endocrinology, 80*, 41–46.

Ghimire, N., & Rao, A. (2013). Comparative evaluation of the influence of television advertisements on children and caries prevalence. *Global Health Action*. https://doi.org/10.3402/gha.v6i0.20066.

Gupta, R., Rastogi, P., & Arora, S. (2006). Low obesity and high undernutrition prevalence in lower socioeconomic status school girls: A double jeopardy. *Human Ecology, 14*, 120–132.

Gupta, D. K., Shah, P., Misra, A., Bharadwaj, S., Gulati, S., Gupta, N., et al. (2011). Secular trends in prevalence of overweight and obesity from 2006 to 2009 in urban Asian Indian adolescents aged 14-17 years. *Plos One, 6*(*2*), e17221. https://doi.org/10.1371/journal.pone.0017221.

Gupta, S., Kalra, S., Kaushik, J. S., & Gupta, P. (2017). Content of food advertising for young adolescents on television. *Indian Journal of Community Medicine: Official Publication of Indian Association of Preventive & Social Medicine, 42*(1), 43–45. https://doi.org/10.4103/0970-0218.199800.

Haboubi, G. J., & Shaikh, R. B. (2009). A comparison of the nutritional status of adolescents from selected schools of South India and UAE: A cross-sectional study. *Indian Journal of Community Medicine, 34*, 108–111.

Harinarayan, C. V., Ramalakshmi, T., Prasad, U. V., Sudhakar, D., Srinivasarao, P. V., Sarma, K. V., & Kumar, E. G. (2007). High prevalence of low dietary calcium, high phytate consumption, and vitamin D deficiency in healthy south Indians. *American Journal of Clinical Nutrition, 85*, 1062–1067.

Herbst, C. A., Menon, K. C., Ferguson, E. L., Thomson, C. D., Bailey, K., Gray, A. R., Zodpey, S., Saraf, A., Das, P. K., & Skeaff, S. A. (2014). Dietary and non-dietary factors associated with serum zinc in Indian women. *Biological Trace Elements Research, 161*, 38–47. https://doi.org/10.1007/s12011-014-0090-9.

International Institute for Population Sciences (IIPS) and Macro International. (2005). *National Family Health Survey (NFHS-3), India, 2005–06*. Mumbai: IIPS.

International Institute for Population Sciences (IIPS) and Macro International. (2007). *National Family Health Survey (NFHS-3), India, 2005–06*. Mumbai: IIPS.

International Institute for Population Sciences (IIPS) and Macro International. (2015). *National Family Health Survey (NFHS-4), India, 2015–16*. Mumbai: IIPS.

International Institute for Population Sciences (IIPS) and Macro International. (2016). *National Family Health Survey (NFHS-4), India, 2015–16*. Mumbai: IIPS.

Jagadesan, S., Harish, R., Miranda, P., Unnikrishnan, R., Anjana, R. M., & Mohan, V. (2014). Prevalence of overweight and obesity among school children and adolescents in Chennai. *Indian Pediatrics, 51*, 544–549.

Jeemon, P., Prabhakaran, D., Mohan, V., Thankappan, K. R., Joshi, P. P., Ahmed, F., SSIP Investigators, et al. (2009). Double burden of underweight and overweight among children (10-19 years of age) of employees working in Indian industrial units. *National Medical Journal of India, 22*, 172–176.

Johnson, A. R., Balasubramanya, B., Jaimol, S., Shaiby, S., Gifty, S., & Britto, R. D. (2015). Body image perception and nutritional status of adolescents in a school in rural South India. *Journal of the Indian Association of Child and Adolescent Mental Health, 11(4)*, 260–278.

Kandpal, E. (2011). *Three essays on investments in child welfare in India*. IDEALS. University of Illinois at Urbana Champagne. https://www.ideals.illinois.edu/handle/2142/26327. Accessed on 15 November, 2016.

Kapil, U., Singh, P., Pathak, P., Dwivedi, S. N., & Bhasin, S. (2002). Prevalence of obesity amongst affluent adolescent school children in Delhi. *Indian Pediatrics, 39*, 449–452.

Kapil, U., Toteja, G. S., Rao, S., & Pandey, R. M. (2011). Zinc deficiency amongst adolescents in Delhi. *Indian Pediatrics, 48*, 981–982.

Katona, P., & Katona-Apte, J. (2008). The interaction between nutrition and infection. *Clinical Infectious Diseases, 46*, 1582–1588.

Kaushal, N., & Muchomba, F. (2013). How consumer price subsidies affect nutrition. *World Development, 74*, 25–42.

Kochar, A. (2005). Can targeted food programs improve nutrition? An empirical analysis of India's public distribution system. *Economic Development and Cultural Change., 54(1)*, 203–235.

Kotian, M. S., Kumar, G. S., & Kotian, S. S. (2010). Prevalence and determinants of overweight and obesity among adolescent school children of South Karnataka, India. *Indian Journal of Community Medicine, 35*, 176–178.

Krishna, J., & Mishra, C. P. (2013). Correlates of nutritional deficiency among urban adolescent girls of Varanasi. *Indian Journal of Preventive Social Medicine, 44*(1–2). http://medind.nic.in/ibl/t13/i1/iblt13i1p102.pdf.

Krishnamurthy, P., Pathania, V., & Tandon, S. (2014). Public distribution system reforms and consumption in Chhattisgarh: A comparative empirical analysis. *Economic & Political Weekly, 49*, 74–81.

Kristjansson, B., Petticrew, M., MacDonald, B., Krasevec, J., Janzen, L., Greenhalgh, T., Wells, G.A., MacGowan, J., Farmer, A.P., Shea, B., Mayhew, A., Tugwell, P., & Welch, V. (2007). School feeding for improving the physical and psychosocial health of disadvantaged students. Cochrane Database of Systematic Reviews, Issue 1. Art. No: CD004676. https://doi.org/10.1002/14651858.CD004676.pub2.

Laxmaiah, A., Nagalla, B., Vijayaraghavan, K., & Nair, M. (2007). Factors affecting prevalence of overweight among 12 to 17 year-old urban adolescents in Hyderabad, India. *Obesity, 15*, 1384–1390.

Lokshin, M., Das Gupta, M., Gragnolati, M., & Ivaschenko.O. (2005). Improving child nutrition: the integrated child development services in India. *Development and Change, 36(4)*, 613–640.

Lone, M. A., & Ganesan, P. (2016). Health and nutritional status of orphan children's living in orphanages with special reference to district Anantnag of Jammu and Kashmir. *The International Journal of Indian Psychology, 3(2)*, 163–169.

Maliye, C., Deshmukh, P., Gupta, S., Kaur, S., Mehendale, A., & Garg, B. (2010). Nutrient intake amongst rural adolescent girls of Wardha. *Indian Journal of Community Medicine, 35*, 400–402.

Maneesh, P. (2015). Mid day meals and food security among children: Assuring nutritional security of Tamil Nadu. *Indian Journal of Economics and Development, 3*(9), http://ijed.informaticspublishing.com/index.php/ijed/article/view/84366/65100

Maheshwar, M., & Vijayapushpam, T. (2014). A current appraisal of health and nutrition related claims in Indian children' television food advertisements. *Journal of Social Science Studies, 1*(2), 125–135.

Marwaha, R. K., Tandon, N., Reddy, D. R., Aggarwal, R., Singh, R., Sawhney, R. C., Saluja, B., Ganie, M. A., & Singh, S. (2005). Vitamin D and bone mineral density status of healthy schoolchildren in northern India. *American Journal of Clinical Nutrition, 82*, 477–482.

Marwaha, R. K., Puri, S., Tandon, N., Dhir, S., Agarwal, N., Bhadra, K., & Saini, N. (2011). Effects of sports training & nutrition on bone mineral density in young Indian healthy females. *Indian Journal of Medical Research, 134*, 307–313.

Mathur, M., Bhargava, R., Benipal, R., Luthra, N., Basu, S., Kaur, J., & Chavan, B. S. (2007). Dietary habits and nutritional status in mentally retarded children and adolescents: A study from North Western India. *Journal of the Indian Association of Child Adolescent Mental Health, 3(2)*, 18–20.

Menon, K. C., Skeaff, S. A., Thomson, C. D., Gray, A. R., Ferguson, E. L., Zodpey, S., Saraf, A., Das, P. K., Toteja, G. S., & Pandav, C. S. (2011). Concurrent micronutrient deficiencies are prevalent in nonpregnant rural and tribal women from central India. *Nutrition, 27(4)*, 496–502. https://doi.org/10.1016/j.nut.2010.02.012.

Ministry of Women and Child Development, Government of India. (1993). *National nutrition policy*. http://wcd.nic.in/sites/default/files/nnp_0.pdf. Accessed on 23rd August, 2016.

Mishra, S. (2002). National support to Primary Education (Mid Day Meal Programme) in Orissa-It's Impact on Enrollment, Attendance, Retention and Drop outs among School going Children. Vision 2020, NCDS, Bhubaneswar.

Mondala, P. R., Sadaruddin, B., & Kaushik, B. (2012). Gender discrimination in under nutrition with mediating factors among Bengalee school children from Eastern India. *Journal of Comparative Human Biology, 63*, 126–135.

Muthayya, S., Rah, J. H., Sugimoto, J. D., et al. (2013). The global hidden hunger indices and maps: An advocacy tool for action. *PLoS One, 8*, e67860. https://doi.org/10.1371/journal.pone.0067860.

Nambiar, V. S., & Desai, R. (2012). Positive and negative deviant behaviors affecting the midday meal programme (MDMP) in government aided primary schools of an urban Indian city: causes, consequences. *International Journal of Biomedical Research and Analysis, 3(3)*, 1–10.

Nambiar, V. S., & Desai, R. (2013). Behaviour change communication strategies for improvement of midday meal in urban Vadodara-western India. *Universal Journal of Pharmacy, 2*(2), 111–117.

Nambiar, V., Desai, R., Patel, N., & Roy, K. (2012a). Mapping the functioning of midday meal programme in schools of rural Vadodara and its impact on the nutritional status of the children. *Journal of Pure and Applied Sciences, 20*, 72–78.

Nambiar, V. S., Nithya, S., & Pandit, N. (2012b). Strengthening the MidDay Meal Programme (MDMP) with non-pharmaceutical measures: Role of dietary diversification and nutrition communication IJPI's. *Journal of Hospital and Clinical Pharmacy, 3*, 11–15.

National Institute of Nutrition. (2011). *Dietary guidelines for Indians: A manual*. Hyderabad: Indian Council of Medical Research.

National Nutrition Monitoring Bureau. (2012). Technical report no. 26. http://nnmbindia.org/1_NNMB_Third_Repeat_Rural_Survey_Technicl.Report_26.pdf. Accessed on 25 September, 2016.

Nawab, T., Khan, Z., Khan, I. M., & Ansari, M. A. (2014). Influence of behavioral determinants on the prevalence of overweight and obesity among school going adolescents of Aligarh. *Indian Journal of Public Health, 58*, 121–124.

Padmapriyadarsini, C., Shobana, M., Lakshmi, M., Beena, T., & Swaminathan, S. (2016). Undernutrition & tuberculosis in India: Situation analysis & the way forward. *Indian Journal of Medical Research, 144*, 11–20. https://doi.org/10.4103/0971-5916.193278.

Pandav, C. S., Yadav, K., Srivastava, R., Pandav, R., & Karmarkar, M. G. (2013). Iodine deficiency disorders (IDD) control in India. *The Indian Journal of Medical Research, 138*(3), 418–433.

Patel, P., Patel, P., Chiplonkar, S., Khadilkar, A., & Patel, A. (2016). Effect of mid-day meal on nutritional status of adolescents: A cross-sectional study from Gujarat. *Indian Journal of Child Health, 3*, 203–207.

Pathak, P., Kapil, U., Kumar, K. S., Nand, D. S., & Singh, R. (2003). Magnitude of zinc deficiency among nulliparous nonpregnant women in a rural community of Haryana State, India. *Food Nutrition Bulletin, 24*, 368–371.

Pednekar, M. S. (2008). Association of body mass index with all-cause and cause-specific mortality: Findings from a prospective cohort study in Mumbai (Bombay), India. *International Journal of Epidemiology, 37*, 524–535.

Pfeiffer, C. M., Johnson, C. L., Jain, R. B., et al. (2007). Trends in blood folate and vitamin B-12 concentrations in the United States, 1988–2004. *American Journal of Clinical Nutrition, 86*, 718–727.

Planning and Evaluation Organization. (2005). *Performance evaluation of targeted public distribution system*. New Delhi: Government of India.

Poobalan, A., & Aucott, L. (2016). Obesity among Young adults in developing countries: A systematic overview. *Current Obesity Reports, 5*, 2–13.

Puri, S., Marwaha, R. K., Agarwal, N., Tandon, N., Agarwal, R., Grewal, K., Reddy, D. H., & Singh, S. (2008). Vitamin D status of apparently healthy schoolgirls from two different socioeconomic strata in Delhi: Relation to nutrition and lifestyle. *British Journal of Nutrition, 99*, 876–882.

Raj, M. (2009). Dynamics of growth and weight transitions in a pediatric cohort from India. *Nutrition Journal, 8*, 55.

Raj, M., & Kumar, R. K. (2010). Obesity in children & adolescents. *Indian Journal of Medical Research, 132(5)*, 598–607.

Ramachandran, A., Snehalatha, C., Vinitha, R., Thayyil, M., Kumar, C. K. S., Sheeba, L., et al. (2002). Prevalence of overweight in urban Indian adolescent school children. *Diabetes Research Clinical Practica, 57*, 185–190.

Rani, M. A., & Sathiyasekaran, B. W. C. (2013). behavioural determinants for obesity: A cross-sectional study among urban adolescents in India. *Journal of Preventive Medicine & Public Health, 46*, 192–200. https://doi.org/10.3961/jpmph.2013.46.4.192.

Rani, M. A., Shriraam, V., Zachariah, R., Harries, A. D., Satyanarayana, S., Tetali, S., Anchala, R., Muthukumar, D., & Sathiyasekaran, B. W. C. (2013). Does a nutrition education programme change the knowledge and practice of healthy diets among high school adolescents in Chennai, India? *Health Education Journal, 72(6)*, 733–741.

Rao, T. V. R. K., & Vijay, T. (2006). Malnutrition and anemia in tribal pediatric population of Purnia district. *Indian Pediatrics, 43*, 181–182.

Rao, V. G., Aggrawal, M. C., Yadav, R., Das, S. K., Sahare, L. K., Bondley, M. K., et al. (2003). Intestinal parasitic infections, anaemia and undernutrition among tribal adolescents of Madhya Pradesh. *Indian Journal of Community Medicine, 28*, 26–29.

Rao, D. R., Vijayapushpam, T., Rao, G. M. S., Antony, G. M., & Sarma, K. V. R. (2007a). Dietary habits and effect of two different educational tools on nutrition knowledge of school going adolescent girls in Hyderabad, India. *European Journal of Clinical Nutrition, 61*, 1081–1085.

Rao, S., Kanade, A., & Kelkar, R. (2007b). Blood pressure among overweight adolescents from urban school children in Pune, India. *European Journal of Clinical Nutrition, 61*, 633–641.

Ray, S., & Ray, I. A. (2011). Role and effectiveness of public distribution system in assuring food security in India: An appraisal. *Journal of Economics and Sustainable Development, 2(4)*, 238–252.

Saijhee, A. (2003). *Child nutrition and poverty in South India-Noon meals in Tamil Nadu*. Concept, New Delhi.

Saxena, N.C. (2003). *Food assistance programme and their role in allocating poverty and hunger in India*. www.righttofood.com. Accessed 21st August, 2016.

Seena, M., & Ramadas, S. V. (2002). Eating habits of young children with Down syndrome. *Indian Journal of Nutrition & Dietetics, 39*, 311–320.

Semba, R. D. (2003). Iron-deficiency anemia and the cycle of poverty among human immunodeficiency virus-infected women in the inner city. *Clinical Infectious Diseases, 37*(Suppl 2), S105–S111.

Sethy, P. G. S., Bulliyya, G., Mallick, G., Swain, B. K., & Kar, S. K. (2007). Iodine deficiency in urban slums of Bhubaneswar. *Indian Journal of Pediatrics, 74(10)*, 917–921.

Shah, S. R., Tullu, M. S., & Kamat, J. R. (2005). Clinical profile of pediatric HIV infection from India. *Archives of Medical Research, 36(1)*, 24–31.

Shah, P., Misra, A., Gupta, N., Hazra, D. K., Gupta, R., Seth, P., Agarwal, A., Gupta, A. K., Jain, A., et al. (2010). Improvement in nutrition-related knowledge and behaviour of urban Asian Indian school children: findings from the 'Medical education for children/Adolescents for Realistic prevention of obesity and diabetes and for healthy ageing' (MARG) intervention study. *British Journal of Nutrition, 104*, 427–436.

Shah, J. S., Patel, P. K., & Patel, B. (2013). Determinants of overweight and obesity among school children in Mehsana District. *Annals of Tropical Medicine and Public Health, 6*(4), 408–412.

Shalini, C. N., Murthy, N. S., Shalini, S., Dinesh, R., Shivaraj, N. S., & Suryanarayana, S. P. (2014). Comparison of nutritional status of rural and urban school students receiving midday meals in schools of Bengaluru, India: A cross sectional study. *Journal of Postgraduate Medicine, 60*, 118–122.

Shet, A., Mehta, S., Rajagopalan, N., Dinakar, C., Ramesh, E., Samuel, N. M., Indumathi, C. K., Fawzi, W. W., & Kurpad, A. V. (2009). Anemia and growth failure among HIV-infected children in India: a retrospective analysis. *BMC Pediatrics, 9*, 37. https://doi.org/10.1186/1471-2431-9-37.

Sidhu, S., Marwah, G., & Prabhjot. (2005). Prevalence of overweight and obesity among the affluent adolescent school children of Amritsar, Punjab. *Collegium Antropologicum, 1*, 53–55.

Sinha, A. (2016). *Rapid assessment of integrated child development scheme in Delhi*. HDBI Project. Delhi Government. Available at: http://www.ihdindia.org/hdidelhi/pdf/icds_report.pdf. Accessed on 10th September.

Sivagurunathan, C., Umadevi, R., Rama, R., & Gopalakrishnan, S. (2015). Adolescent health: Present status and its related programmes in India. Are we in the right direction? *Journal of Clinical and Diagnostic Research, 9(3)*, LE01–LE06.

Stigler, M. H. (2011). Weight-related concerns and weight-control behaviors among overweight adolescents in Delhi, India: A cross-sectional study. *International Journal of Behavioral Nutrition & Physical Activity, 8*, 9.

Thankachan, P., Muthayya, S., Walczyk, T., Kurpad, A. V., & Hurrell, R. F. (2007). An analysis of the etiology of anemia and iron deficiency in young women of low socioeconomic status in Bangalore, India. *Food Nutrition Bulletin, 28(3)*, 328–336.

Tharkar, S., & Viswanathan, V. (2009). Impact of socioeconomic status on prevalence of overweight and obesity among children and adolescents in urban India. *The Open Obesity Journal, 1*, 9–14.

Toteja, G. S., Singh, P., Dhillon, B. S., & Saxena, B. N. (2002). Vitamin A deficiency disorders in 16 districts of India. *Indian Journal of Pediatrics, 69*, 603–605.

Toteja, G. S., Singh, P., Dhillon, B. S., Saxena, B. N., Ahmed, F. U., Singh, R. P., Prakash, B., Vijayaraghavan, K., Singh, Y., Rauf, A., Sarma, U. C., Gandhi, S., Behl, L., Mukherjee, K., Swami, S. S., Meru, V., Chandra, P., & Chandrawati, M. U. (2006). Prevalence of anemia among pregnant women and adolescent girls in 16 districts of India. *Food Nutrition Bulletin, 27(4)*, 311–315.

UN ACC/SCN. (2000). *Fourth report on the World nutrition situation: Nutrition throughout the life cycle*. Geneva: ACC/SCN in Collaboration with IFPRI.

UN Department of Economic and Social Affairs. (2004). *World Youth Report 2003: The global situation of young people*. New York: UN.

UNFPA. (2003). *State of the World population 2003*. http://www.unfpa.org/swop. Accessed on 18 August, 2016.

UNFPA. (2014). *State of the world population UNFPA*: New York. http://www.unfpa.org/swop. Accessed on 18th August, 2016.

UNICEF. (2013). *Improving child nutrition: The achievable imperative for global progress*. New York.

United Nations Children's Fund. (2006). *Progress on children*. https://www.unicef.org/progressforchildren/2006n4/undernutritiondefinition.html. Accessed on: 26th April, 2017.

Unnikrishnan, A. G., Kalra, S., Sahay, R. K., Bantwal, G., John, M., & Tewari, N. (2013). Prevalence of hypothyroidism in adults: An epidemiological study in eight cities of India. *Indian Journal of Endocrinology and Metabolism, 17(4)*, 647–652.

Vikram, N. K., Tandon, N., Misra, A., Srivastava, M. C., Pandey, R. M., Mithal, A., et al. (2006). Correlates of Type 2 diabetes mellitus in children, adolescents and young adults in north India: A multisite collaborative case control study. *Diabetes Medicine, 23*, 293–298.

Wasnik, V., Rao, B. S., & Rao, D. (2012). A study of the health status of 17. Early adolescent girls residing in social welfare hostels in Vizianagaram district of Andhra Pradesh state, India. *International Journal of Collaborative Research on Internal Medicine & Public Health*. http://www.iomcworld.com/ijcrimph/files/v04-n01-07.pdf

Welch, R. M. (2002). The impact of mineral nutrients in food crops on global human health. *Plant and Soil, 247*, 83–90.

World Food Program. (2013). *State of School Feeding Programme*. http://www.wfp.org/content/state-school-feeding-worldwide-2013. Accessed on 20 August, 2016.

World Health Organization (2001). *Iron deficiency anaemia: Assessment, prevention and control, a guide for programme managers*. Geneva: World Health Organization. Accessed on 20 January, 2017.

World Health Organization. (2005). *Adolescent health*. https://www.who.int/maternal_child_adolescent/adolescence/en/. Accessed on 18th August, 2016.

World Health Organization. (2009). *Global prevalence of vitamin A deficiency in populations at risk 1995-2005: WHO global database on vitamin A deficiency*. Geneva: World Health Organization.

Zimmermann, M. B. (2009). Iodine deficiency in pregnancy and the effects of maternal iodine supplementation on the offspring: A review. *American Journal of Clinical Nutrition, 89*, 668S–672S.

Zimmermann, M. B., Jooste, P. L., & Pandav, C. S. (2008). Iodine-deficiency disorders. *Lancet, 372*, 1251–2162.

Chapter 3
Adolescent and Youth Mental Health in India: Status and Needs

Chetna Duggal and Lamia Bagasrawala

Abstract Adolescence and youth are important developmental stages marking the transition from childhood to adulthood. The prevalence of psychological disorders among adolescents and young individuals is on the rise. However, the data on psychological disorders among adolescents and youth is not extensively available and consolidated. The chapter therefore aims to provide comprehensive information about mental health needs of adolescents and youth in India as identified by existing research, as well as by experts in the field. The chapter will begin with an understanding of adolescence and youth as significant developmental stages, followed by an overview of the status of mental health of adolescents and youth in India through a meta-analytical desk review of epidemiological studies over the last 15 years, highlighting the prevalence of psychological disorders and associated risk and protective factors. This will be corroborated with inputs received from mental health professionals and experts consulted as part of the study. Cross-cutting issues like stigma, discrimination and vulnerable populations will be discussed alongside. The chapter concludes with developing a proposal for future research and recommendations to enhance adolescent and youth mental health in India.

Keywords Adolescents and youth · Mental health · Psychological disorders · Adolescent mental health · Youth mental health

Adolescence and youth are periods of great possibilities and opportunities characterised by rapid physical, cognitive and emotional development. Individuals in this age group are often seen as being curious, innovative and engaged (Kleinert and Horton 2016) and demonstrating the potential to challenge existing conditions and initiating and giving momentum to change.

C. Duggal (✉)
School of Human Ecology, Tata Institute of Social Sciences, Mumbai, India
e-mail: chetna.d@tiss.edu

L. Bagasrawala
Tata Institute of Social Sciences, Mumbai, India

S. Bharat, G. Sethi (eds.), *Health and Wellbeing of India's Young People*,
https://doi.org/10.1007/978-981-13-6593-5_3

The World Health Organization (WHO) identifies adolescence as a period of "tremendous growth and potential", as well as that of "considerable risk" (WHO 2016). It is important to recognise the possible concerns and problems that may arise during this period of transition and development. Mental health problems have been reported to account for a large proportion of the burden of disease on young people globally, with depression being the highest contributor in the age group of 15–19 years (UNICEF 2011). Suicide is the second leading cause of death among young individuals between the ages 15 and 29 years globally (World Health Organization 2014). Thus, there is an urgent need to invest in adolescent and youth mental health.

The onset of many adult mental health disorders is often traced to adolescence and teenage years (Jones 2013). Some of these problems, like the use of psychoactive substances and alcohol, may begin as lifestyle experiments for peer acceptance during adolescence (Nowinski 1990) and may later present as a problem during youth, while others like psychosis may have their onset in youth, often preceded by an unidentified phase of prodromal symptoms during childhood and adolescence (Stevens et al. 2014). It is therefore important to identify the mental health needs of adolescents and youth in order to ensure a smooth and healthy transition into adulthood.

Mental health of adolescents and youth has been identified as a significant public health challenge globally and an important area of action to promote adolescent and youth development (UNFPA 2013; UNICEF 2011). In his message on the International Youth Day 2014, UN Secretary-General Ban Ki-moon highlighted the need to create awareness about and invest in mental health of young people. He identified the role of education in reducing stigma and encouraged open discussions about mental health. He concluded his message by saying, "As we mark International Youth Day 2014, let us enable youth with mental health conditions to realize their full potential, and let us show that mental health matters to us all" (United Nations Development Programme 2014). The need for strategic interventions to enhance the mental health of adolescents and youth and address psychological disorders among them is therefore crucial and urgent.

3.1 The Indian Context

India has the world's largest adolescent and youth population, according to the Census of India 2011. Adolescents and youth between the ages of 10 years and 24 years constitute 30.12% of the total population (Census of India 2011). This large section of the population can contribute to the economic and social development of the nation by entering the productive workforce, helping India achieve its "demographic dividend", only if their health and wellbeing needs are fulfilled. Therefore, for India to continue on its growth path, it is important to identify the health risks and mental health concerns of this population and work towards improving their health status to enhance their life satisfaction, ensure productivity at work, and manage future health expenditure (Chandrasekhar et al. 2006).

3.2 Methods

This chapter is based on a desk review of available published and unpublished documents, reports, journal research papers and policy and programme manuals, along with inputs and insights received from expert field practitioners and stakeholders through interviews and consultations.

An extensive search of academic literature was conducted across search engines like PubMed, JSTOR, Sage, Wiley Online Library, ScienceDirect and Google Scholar and by accessing and requesting papers from Research Gate and Acdemia. edu. Key search words included, but were not limited to, "psychiatry, epidemiology, adolescents, youth, children, mental health problems, India and prevalence". Studies conducted in India on adolescents and youth between January 2001 and August 2016 were included.

For the purpose of this chapter, all individuals between the ages of 10 years and 18 years are considered as adolescents and those between the ages of 19 years and 24 years as youth. A total of 17 research studies were reviewed and critically analysed for the chapter, of which 3 are review studies and the remaining provide quantitative data in terms of prevalence rates and percentages. This chapter includes review of studies of prevalence of mental health concerns among adolescents only. Some studies for specific disorders which were identified as significant by experts but not included in the 17 studies reviewed have also been included. Epidemiological studies specific to only youth are not available for the selected time period.

Studies conducted in schools, colleges, community settings and health centres were included, while studies conducted in clinical or psychiatric units have been excluded from this review. This is done to provide an understanding of the prevalence rates in the general population and not specific to clinical populations or those reporting distress or seeking treatment. Qualitative studies reporting prevalence through personal accounts of individuals are not available for this period. In addition to research papers published in peer-reviewed journals, reports published by the United Nations Population Fund (UNFPA) and World Health Organization (WHO), as well as reviews and reports published for the Ministry of Health and Family Welfare, Government of India, were also reviewed. Handbooks and implementation guideline manuals of the national-level programme Rashtriya Kishor Swasthya Karyakram (RKSK) were also reviewed.

The desk review and analysis was supplemented with information received from in-depth interviews and consultations with experts. A series of ten interviews were conducted over the phone and in person, with field practitioners, government officials and researchers working in the area of adolescent and youth mental health. In order to receive data on existing psychological disorders among adolescents and youth, with respect to available research in the field and service provisions for the same, a series of eight consultations were conducted in Bangalore with experts from the National Institute of Mental Health and Neurosciences (NIMHANS). A national consultative meet was organised at the Tata Institute of Social Sciences (TISS), Mumbai campus, to bring together experts involved in policy-making, central and state government officials working in the field of adolescent and youth mental health and adolescent and youth leaders. This consultation focused on three broad areas of discussion related to mental health: status and future imperatives for national-level policies, programmatic-level recommendations and exploration of possibilities for adolescent and youth engagement and leadership. The 3.5 hour consultative meet led to a thought-provoking discussion on ways of enhancing adolescent and youth mental health in India.

This chapter presents data from the epidemiological studies, analysed along various sociocultural axes and corroborated with inputs from experts received during the aforementioned interviews and consultations.

3.3 Status of Adolescent and Youth Mental Health in India

In order to understand the prevalence of psychological disorders among adolescents, a review of epidemiological research was conducted. This section will begin by presenting and reviewing the Census 2011 and National Sample Survey Office (NSSO) 2002 data on prevalence of mental illness and psychological disorders among adolescents in India. This national data will be followed by presenting prevalence rates recorded in one of the most recent large-scale mental health surveys conducted by NIMHANS. After a brief review of the above data, prevalence rates of psychological disorders and psychosocial concerns among adolescents from the 17 epidemiological studies reviewed for this chapter will be discussed. Table 3.1 presents details of these studies conducted across different regions and settings within India.

3.3.1 National-Level Data on Prevalence of Psychological Disorders Among Adolescents in India

In India, the only prevalence rates of psychological disorders among adolescents at the national level are available from the Census (2011) and the NSSO (2002). The NSSO 2002 was the first time the NSSO included mental illness within its purview. The survey identified age as a significant predictor of mental illness and found that prevalence of mental illness increases with age (Lakhan and Ekúndayò 2015). The NSSO data found the prevalence of mental illness increasing from 0.54 persons per 1000 in the age group 10–14 years, 0.82 per 1000 in the age group 15–19 years to 1.01 per 1000 for those between the ages 20 and 24 years. The study therefore found age to be a strong predictor of mental illness in both urban and rural populations (Lakhan and Ekúndayò 2015). However, since the NSSO does not mention the tools used for the study and does not provide the criteria used to define mental illness, it is important to corroborate this data with findings from other epidemiological studies.

Table 3.1 Epidemiological studies reviewed to assess prevalence rates of mental health concerns among adolescents arranged chronologically

Sr. No.	Year	Authors	Sample size (N)	Location	Setting	Age of sample	Tools/instruments used	Prevalence rate	Mental health concerns identified
01	2001	Mishra and Sharma	1097 students	New Delhi	Students of classes 8–12 from 3 schools	12–18 years	Youth Self-Report 1989 + self-designed questionnaire	13.76%	Internalising problems most common, followed by problems that were neither internalising nor externalising followed by externalising problems; anxiety/depression highest at 10.3% followed by social problems at 5%, aggressive behaviour syndrome at 4.4% and somatic syndrome at 4.38% , attention problems (4.1%) and withdrawn behaviour (2.55%)
02	2001	Verma, Singh, Gupta and Gupta	957	Ludhiana		09–11 years	Stage 1: Rutter B Stage 2: Psychiatric interview	14.63% as detected in Stage 1, 45.5% from both Stages 1 and 2	In Stage 1, of the 141 children showing difficulties on Rutter B – 59.6%, antisocial; 27%, neurotic; 13%, presenting mixed symptoms

(continued)

Table 3.1 (continued)

Sr. No.	Year	Authors	Sample size (N)	Location	Setting	Age of sample	Tools/instruments used	Prevalence rate	Mental health concerns identified
03	2003	Gaur, Vohra, Subash and Khurana	800	Rohtak	Rural and urban field practice areas of Dept. of SPM, PGIMS	6–14 years	Phase 1:CPMS – Hindi Version, Phase 2: DISC	16.50%	Conduct disorder, 4.5%; MR, 3.25%; anxiety, 2.87%; psychotic symptoms, 1.87%, followed by enuresis, somnambulism, pica, somatisation and depression
04	2005	Rahi, Kumavat, Garg and Singh	620 children	Miraj, Maharashtra	Urban slum	04–14 years	CPMS +schedule for socio-demographic data	16.50%	
05	2005	Srinath et al.	2064	Bangalore	5 urban blocks, 3 urban slums, 3 villages	0–16	ICD-10 criteria; SCL, SDP, CBCL, AM, CBQ, FTN, PIS, SIS, DISC, VSMS, BKT, SLD battery, CGAS, PE proforma	12.5% in age group 0–16 years	In 04–16 years – enuresis 6.2%, specific phobias 2.9%, hyperkinetic disorders 1.6%, stuttering 1.5% and oppositional defiant disorder (ODD) 0.9%
06	2007	Ahmad, Khalique, Khan and Amir	390 students	Aligarh	Rural and urban schools	10–19 years	Stage 1, psychosocial history and screening using Y-PSC; Stage 2, those with suspected psychosocial problems referred to psychiatrist for diagnosis as per ICD 10 criteria	17.90%	Educational difficulties, 17.4%; substance use difficulties, 13.3%; conduct disorders, 9.2%; anxiety 3.8%; and depression, 3.1%

07	2008	Pillai, Patel, Cardozo, Goodman, Weiss and Andrew	2048	Goa		12–16	DSM- IV criteria using the DAWBA +structured interviews for socio-demographic data	1.81%	Anxiety disorders were the most common (1.0%), followed by depressive disorders (0.5%), behavioural disorders (0.4%) and attention-deficit hyperactivity disorder (ADHD) (0.2%)
08	2009	Arun and Chavan	2402 students	Chandigarh	Students from classes 7–11 from 10 schools		GHQ (Hindi version) for screening psychological problems +Mooney Problem Checklist to assess stress + Suicide Risk Eleven to assess for suicidal ideas	45.80%	
09	2010	Math and Srinivasaraju	Review of existing studies through search of PubMed, NeuroMed, *Indian Journal of Psychiatry* website and MEDLARS using search terms "psychiatry", "prevalence", "community" and "epidemiology" was done along with the manual search of journals and cross-references					Range – 9.5 to 102/1000 population	

(continued)

Table 3.1 (continued)

Sr. No.	Year	Authors	Sample size (N)	Location	Setting	Age of sample	Tools/instruments used	Prevalence rate	Mental health concerns identified
10	2011	Reddy, Biswas and Rao	354 students	Bangalore	High school students from 3 urban schools	11–16 years	Strengths and Difficulties Questionnaire (SDQ)	8.7% had an abnormal SDQ score, and 15.3% had a borderline abnormal SDQ score	Conduct problems, 16.7%; emotional problems, 12.4%; hyperactivity, 12.1%; peer problems, 6.2%
11	2012	Samanta, Mukherjee, Ghosh and Dasgupta	199 students	West Bengal	Students from classes 8 and 9	13–15 years	Self-developed questionnaire		Severe worry hampering studies or work, considering suicide in the last 12 months, feeling lonely, worrying causing difficulties in sleeping and eating
12	2013	Patil, Nagaonkar, Shah and Bhat	257 children	Mumbai	Urban health centre post in an urban slum	05–14 years	Introductory interview for socio-demographic details, diagnostic screening interview for diagnosing psychiatric disorders based on DSM-IV criteria; Stage 1, interviews; Stage2, those fulfilling DSM-IV criteria referred to CGC for psychiatric diagnosis	14.8% (38 cases) psychiatric morbidity, 5.5%, comorbid disorders	Non-organic enuresis, 6.2%; ADHD, 4.3%; conduct disorder, 2.7%; mental retardation, 2.3%

13	2014	Malhotra, S. and Patra, B. N	16 community-based studies on 14594 children and adolescents + 07 school-based studies on 5687 children and adolescents					Prevalence of child and adolescent psychiatric disorders in community, 6.46%, in school, 23.33%	
14	2014	Singh, S. and Gururaj, G.	Review of nine studies to assess prevalence rates of common mental disorders			15–24		2.22%	
15	2015	NIMHANS	283 children		23 Schools	07–17 years		347 cases of mental health disorders identified (one child having more than one disorder)	20% experienced emotional concerns related to anxiety, adjustment or depression; 32% behavioural problems, ADHD, conduct problems; 27%, learning problems; 18%, developmental disabilities
			62 children		12 PHCs	0–17 years		96 cases diagnosed	Developmental disabilities followed by behavioural problems, emotional problems and learning issues

(continued)

Table 3.1 (continued)

Sr. No.	Year	Authors	Sample size (N)	Location	Setting	Age of sample	Tools/instruments used	Prevalence rate	Mental health concerns identified
16	2016	Bhola, Sathyanarayanan, Rekha, Daniel and Thomas	1087	Bangalore		Mean age 16.4	SDQ	10.1% reported total difficulties level in the abnormal range	Conduct problems most prevalent, 13%; hyperactivity/inattention problems, 12.6%; peer-related problems, 9.4%; emotional symptoms, 9%
17	2016	Chandrashekarappa, S. M., Ramakrishnaiah, N. M., Ram, D. and Manjunath, R.	664	Mysore	Preuniversity and degree college	16–19	MINI 6.0	16%	Major depressive disorder, 37%; panic disorder and social phobia, 15.7%; dysthymia, 12.3%; post-traumatic stress disorder (PTSD), 10%; obsessive-compulsive disorder (OCD), 7.8%; GAD, 6.7%

Note: *CPMS* Childhood Psychopathology Measurement Schedule, *DISC* Diagnostic Interview Schedule for Children, *ICD-10* International Classification of Diseases, *SCL* Screening Checklist, *SDP* socio-demographic proforma, *CBCL* Child Behaviour Checklist, *AM* Additional Module, *CBQ* Children's Behaviour Questionnaire, *FTN* Felt Treatment Needs, *PIS* Parent Interview Schedule, *SIS* structured interview schedule, *VSMS* Vineland Social Maturity Scale, *BKT* Binet-Kamat test, *SLD* Specific Learning Disability Battery, *CGAS* Children's Global Assessment Scale, *PE* proforma Physical Examination proforma, *Y-PSC* Youth Report of Paediatric Symptom Checklist, *DSM-IV Diagnostic and Statistical Manual-IV*, *DAWBA* Development and Well-Being Assessment, *GHQ* General Health Questionnaire, *CGC* Child Guidance Clinic, *MINI* Mini-International Neuropsychiatric Interview

Table 3.2 Disorder-specific studies reviewed for this chapter arranged chronologically

Sr. no.	Year	Authors	Sample size (N)	Location	Setting	Age of sample	Tools/instruments used	Prevalence rate
01	2013	Goel, Subramanyam and Kamath,	987 boys and girls	Mumbai	Urban – 3 colleges	16–18 years	Young's Internet Addiction Test (1998)	0.7% – addicted to the Internet 24.8% – likely to become addicted 74.5% – engaging in moderate usage of the Internet
02	2016	Jaisoorya et. al	7560 boys and girls	Bangalore	73 schools	12–19 years	Checklist for socio-demographic data; the Alcohol, Smoking and Substance Involvement Screening Test (ASSIST); Kessler's Psychological Distress Scale (K10); and other tools for other variables	Prevalence of alcohol use – 15% Mean age of onset of alcohol use – 13.6years
03	2016	Sharma and Chaudhary	110 males	Meerut	Slums	12–16 years	Self-designed questionnaire	46.36% – using substances 8.18% – showed signs of addiction to drugs
04	2017	Jhala and Sharma	1657 boys and girls	Vadodara, Gujarat	10 schools (urban and rural)	13–19 years	Young's Internet Addiction Test (1998)	44.8%, average users of the Internet; 14.6%, above average users; 0.5%, significantly above average users

The Census data on mental disability includes two areas of focus – mental retardation (now called intellectual disability) and mental illness, under "mental disability". It lists down a few criteria to define mental illness and mental retardation. While these include criteria of different mental disorders covered in the *Diagnostic and Statistical Manual*, the definitions are not comprehensive. According to the Census (2011), over four lakh adolescents between 10 and 19 years of age and over three lakh individuals in the ages 20–29 years are living with mental retardation in the country. The Census (2011) also showed that over two lakh adolescents and young individuals between the ages 10 and 29 years have a mental illness. The figures suggested that 0.17% of India's adolescents have mental retardation and 0.04% have a mental illness. The data also showed that 0.15% of India's youth between the ages 20 and 29 years have mental retardation and 0.05% of youth have a mental illness.

In addition to the NSSO (2002) and Census (2011), the NIMHANS National Mental Health Survey (2016), conducted in 12 states in India, was another source of national-level data on prevalence of mental illness in India. The survey assessed the prevalence of psychological disorders across adolescents between ages 13 and 17 years from four states, using the Mini-International Neuropsychiatric Interview (MINI). According to this survey, the prevalence of psychological disorders was reported as 7.3% among adolescents in the age group 13–17 years with depression, agoraphobia, intellectual disability, autism spectrum disorder, anxiety and psychotic disorders being most common. The summary report of the survey also mentioned data from a study of adolescents and youth in Himachal Pradesh between the ages 15 and 24 years, conducted by NIMHANS (Gururaj et al. 2014) which reported depression (6.9%), anxiety, (15.5%), tobacco (7.6%), alcohol (7.2%) and suicidal ideation (5.5%) as common mental health problems requiring immediate intervention.

This data shows that prevalence of psychological disorders among Indian adolescents in urban and rural areas is high and requires urgent attention. Section 3.3.2 will review 17 epidemiological studies along with some disorder-specific studies to understand the mental health concerns prevalent among adolescents across different sociocultural contexts.

3.3.2 Review of Epidemiological Studies

This section will review the studies mentioned in Table 3.1 along various factors like sampling, age of respondents, tools used for data collection and most prevalent disorders. This will be followed by understanding the findings across three major axes of gender, geographical location and socio-economic correlates.

3.3.2.1 Sampling Across the Studies

As seen in Table 3.1, most studies to assess prevalence of adolescent psychological disorders are conducted in states in southern India like Karnataka (Bhola et al. 2016; Chandrashekarappa et al. 2016; Srinath et al. 2005; Reddy et al. 2011) and Goa (Pillai et al. 2008) and some states in northern India such as Punjab (Arun and Chavan 2009; Verma et al. 2001), Uttar Pradesh (Ahmad et al. 2007) and New Delhi (Mishra and Sharma 2001). Some studies are also conducted in Maharashtra (western India) (Patil et al. 2013; Rahi et al. 2005) and one study in West Bengal (Samanta et al. 2012). Sample sizes vary widely ranging from 62 to 2064, and information on sampling procedures for most studies is unavailable. There is absence of epidemiological data of psychological disorders among adolescents in the north-eastern states of India.

3.3.2.2 Age of Respondents

Most epidemiological studies reviewed do not have commonly defined age ranges. Some studies include adolescents in the ages 10–18 years as part of the larger sample of children, while some include youth between the ages 19 and 24 years as part of the adolescent group. In the studies reviewed, the age of the sample ranges from 0 to 24 years. While findings specific to adolescents between the ages 10 and 19 years are the focus of this chapter, the inconsistency in age group identification and definition results in the variation of prevalence rates reported across various studies.

3.3.2.3 Data Collection Procedures

Most epidemiological studies mainly assess behavioural and emotional aspects of mental health commonly identified as common mental health disorders to severe mental disorders. Of these, most studies assess the prevalence through standardised screening tools such as MINI, General Health Questionnaire, CPMS and Suicide Risk Eleven, among others which define disorders based on the criteria provided in the *International Classification of Diseases* or *Diagnostic and Statistical Manual*. Some studies have also used detailed interview proformas for socio-demographic data. Other studies have used self-reporting measures, as well as checklists to identify prevalence of various psychological disorders among the respondents. Some studies have also used self-designed tools to identify prevalence of psychosocial concerns such as peer problems, interpersonal problems and emotional difficulties that cannot be clinically diagnosed.

3.3.2.4 Prevalence of Different Psychological Disorders

The prevalence of psychological disorders as emerging from the studies reviewed, ranges from 0.20% (National Sample Survey Organisation 2002) to 45.8% (Arun and Chavan 2009). This wide variation in prevalence rates of psychological disorders has also been observed in previously conducted reviews (Bhola and Kapur 2003; Malhotra and Patra 2014; Singh and Gururaj 2014) and can be attributed to the variation in screening tools used across the studies, the differences in sample sizes, age of sample, locations, settings and problems or disorders assessed (Belfer 2005). Variations may also be due to under-reporting and lack of objectivity in defining a "case" or a diagnosable disorder (Math et al. 2007).

In addition to the studies mentioned, prevalence of psychological disorders among adolescents was also studied among those seeking services at the Adolescent Friendly Health Clinics (AFHCs), set up as part of the RKSK program. The prevalence rates in the study were assessed through detailed questionnaires provided to a representative sample of married and unmarried adolescents and youth between the ages 15 and 24 years residing in the 48 villages surrounding the 12 AFHCs identified for the study across the 3 states. The self-report questionnaire was designed in the local language to seek information about the respondent's socio-economic background, mental health concerns experienced in the last 3 months, treatment-seeking patterns, reasons for not seeking treatment, awareness and perceptions of AFHCs, difficulties faced in seeking treatment from these clinics, perceptions about the key health problems and concerns faced by adolescents and youth, etc. This study, conducted in the states of Maharashtra, Jharkhand and Rajasthan, found that 17.5% young men and 25.2% of young women who visited the AFHCs reported experiencing a mental health concern (Santhya et al. 2014).

The review indicates that emotional difficulties are the most commonly experienced psychological disorders among adolescents. Depression (37%) and anxiety-related disorders such as generalised anxiety (6.7%), obsessive-compulsive disorder (7.8%) and panic attacks (15.7%) have been found to be most prevalent among adolescents (Chandrashekarappa et al. 2016) as are feelings of worry and loneliness (Samanta et al. 2012). Conduct disorder was found to be highly prevalent among adolescents across various studies with prevalence rates as high as 16.7% (Reddy et al. 2011), 13% (Bhola et al. 2016) and also 27% (NIMHANS 2015). Adolescents also experience concerns such as attention-deficit hyperactivity disorder (ADHD) with prevalence rates ranging from 0.2% (Pillai et al. 2008) to 4.3% (Patil et al. 2013). The prevalence of other disorders such as oppositional defiant disorder (ODD) (0.9%) (Srinath et al. 2005), psychotic disorders (1.87%) (Gaur et al. 2003), phobias such as social phobia (15.7%) (Chandrashekarappa et al. 2016) and specific phobias (2.9%) (Srinath et al. 2005), somatic symptoms (4.38%) (Mishra and Sharma 2001) and other behavioural disorders (0.4%) (Pillai et al. 2008) is also found to be high among adolescents. In the studies reviewed, peer-related problems has been seen as contributing significantly to difficulties in everyday life, friendships and classroom interactions of adolescents (Bhola et al. 2016; Reddy et al. 2011). The prevalence rates for specific disorders also vary widely across all the studies. The data from these studies do not show any distinct correlational trends between age of respondents and prevalence of specific psychological disorders. This shows that psychological disorders may be influenced by sociocultural contexts and the age of onset may vary depending on biological and psychosocial vulnerability. However, the data from all the studies show that emotional concerns, psychotic symptoms and behavioural concerns are commonly reported psychological disorders among adolescents and youth in India. A few studies have also indicated the presence of comorbid conditions (Mishra and Sharma 2001; Pillai et al. 2008; Patil et al. 2013) such as anxiety and depression and emotional and behavioural concerns.

In addition to depression, anxiety and behavioural problems, substance use is highly prevalent among adolescents and youth (Reddy et al. 2011). The Global Youth Tobacco Survey 2006 (Sinha 2006) showed that 3.8% adolescent students smoke tobacco and 11.9% used smokeless tobacco. In a study of 7560 adolescents in the age group 12–19 years across 73 schools in Bangalore, the prevalence of alcohol use was 15% with the prevalence rates increasing with age (Jaisoorya et al. 2016). The study also found that alcohol use was more common among boys (23.2%) than girls (6.5%). A significant finding was that the mean age of onset of alcohol use was 13.6 years. The study also showed that peer and family influence were strong factors responsible for initiation of alcohol use as reported by the students. Further, the study also found alcohol use to be associated with other mental health problems like drug use, suicidal thoughts and ADHD. This data shows the urgent need to address substance use among school-going adolescents in India. In another study of drug and substance use among slum-dwelling adolescents, it was found that 46.36% of the adolescents were using substances, of which 8.18% showed signs of addiction to drugs (Sharma and Chaudhary 2016). These young individuals were mainly using substances like *ganja*, *gutka*, marijuana, *afeem* and tobacco. This study also found that 5.88% of adolescents used multiple substances. The role of peer influence in initiating substance use was also found in this study. It is important therefore to acknowledge that adolescents across different socio-economic backgrounds are vulnerable to substance use; however, the nature of substances they may use may differ.

Apart from substance addiction, over the last few years, adolescents are also experiencing addiction to electronic gadgets, gaming and the Internet (Wallace 2014). While this has not been included in the studies reviewed as part of the epidemiological review, it is important to highlight as an area requiring attention and intervention. With globalisation and technological advances, the Internet has in fact become a basic necessity. The use of social media is no longer a luxury but a tool to remain connected with those around. In fact, India has recognised this need with its national agenda of digitising all platforms and transactions and making information digitally available to all. In light of such trends, it is extremely important to understand how Internet use is affecting the young population of the nation and its impact on their wellbeing. In a study of 987 adolescents between the ages 16 and 18 years in Mumbai, India, Internet usage was assessed using Young's Internet Addiction Test (1998). The study found that 0.7% of the sample was addicted to the Internet,

24.8% were likely to become addicted and 74.5% were engaging in moderate usage of the Internet (Goel et al. 2013). The same study also found that excessive Internet usage was associated with higher scores on anxiety and depression. In another study of Internet use using Young's Internet Addiction Test among 1657 adolescents between the ages 13 and 19 years from urban and rural areas of Vadodara, Gujarat, it was found that 44.8% of the adolescents were average users of the Internet, 14.6% were above average users and 0.5% were significantly above average users (Jhala and Sharma 2017). Male participants in this study reported using more Internet as compared to their female counterparts. The study also found a linear relationship between Internet usage and age of respondents. Adolescents from urban and rural areas were both found to be using the Internet excessively. These findings indicate the need to address excessive Internet use among adolescents across urban and rural settings under the purview of adolescent mental health and wellbeing. However, as discussed above, given the modern-day requirements of the Internet, it is important to study the purpose of Internet usage along with the extent of use.

While psychotic symptoms and psychosis have not been studied extensively in the studies reviewed, it would be important to discuss the same, as psychosis often has its onset during middle childhood and adolescence and most cases are reported between 15 and 30 years (Srivastava et al. 2014). In a meta-analysis of population-based studies in 2012, the prevalence of psychotic symptoms was found to be as high as 17% among children and adolescents between 9 and 12 years of age and 7.5% among adolescents between the ages 13 and 18 years (Kelleher et al. 2012). While there is significant data on onset and prevalence of psychosis during adolescence globally, there is absence of such national data in India.

Suicide and suicidal ideation have also been found as a significant mental health concern among young adolescents in the country in the studies reviewed. In a study of 199 male adolescents of classes 8 and 9 in urban and rural West Bengal, prevalence of suicidal thoughts was found to be as high as 19.2% among the urban sample and 14.1% among the rural sample (Samanta et al. 2012). In another study of 2404 adolescent students in Chandigarh, 6% reported experiencing suicidal thoughts and 0.39% reported attempting suicide (Arun and Chavan 2009). While this data is specific to certain states, suicide is found to be the leading cause of death among adolescent boys and girls in India (The Lancet 2016). According to the National Crime Records Bureau, suicide rates among adolescents and youth in the age group 15–29 years have been increasing every year and increased from 3.73 to 3.96 per 1,00,000 population between 2002 and 2011 (National Crime Records Bureau Ministry of Home Affairs 2012). According to the WHO report on preventing suicide, India has the highest suicide rate at 35.5% for young individuals in the age group 15–29 years in the world (WHO 2014). The role of academic stressors as one of the leading risk factors for suicide is evident in the high rates of suicides in Kota, India. Kota is the hub of coaching institutes for students seeking admissions to top medical and engineering colleges in India. According to a recent report, 17 student suicides were recorded in 2016 in Kota (Hindustan Times 2017).

The wide range of psychological disorders experienced by adolescents in India and the high prevalence rates present an urgent need to critically review this data and develop a robust plan to address adolescent and youth mental health needs effectively. Experts and practitioners consulted for this review identified depression, substance use, suicide and non-suicidal self-injury as highly prevalent among adolescents and youth. They also mentioned that there was an increasing trend among adolescents and youth to seek professional help for emotional distress and psychological disorders. Experts reported that substance use is reported more among boys, but the prevalence among adolescent girls seems to be increasing too. Adolescents from lower socio-economic backgrounds and young individuals in school report using substances like *gutka*. Psychosis is another major concern among adolescents and youth that was highlighted by experts as requiring critical attention. Exam anxiety, peer pressure, bullying, body image concerns, feeling singled out, sexual experimentation, sexual and physical abuse, relationship issues in family, etc. are also significant psychosocial concerns experienced by adolescents as informed by experts. These problems can continue to persist into adulthood if not identified and addressed during adolescence. It is important therefore to provide mental healthcare services across different levels of care, ranging from universal prevention, selective prevention to specialised intervention, for the different psychological problems experienced by adolescents.

3.3.2.5 Gender and Prevalence of Psychological Disorders

The WHO identifies gender as a significant factor influencing mental health outcomes and treatment. According to the WHO Department of Mental Health and Substance Dependence. (n.d.), "Gender differentially affects the power and control men and women have over these socioeconomic determinants, their access to resources, and their status, roles, options and treatment in society". It is important therefore to understand the role of gender in adolescent mental health needs and outcomes. According to the Census (2011), mental illness is slightly more prevalent in adolescent boys (0.005%) than girls (0.003%). This is congruent with other studies which also report higher prevalence rates for psychological disorders among boys than girls (Patil et al. 2013; Rahi et al. 2005) and significantly so for conduct disorder and psychotic symptoms (Gaur et al. 2003). Researchers suggest that this could merely be a difference of higher reporting. Since young boys are given more preference in the Indian sociocultural context, they also have more access to healthcare services and are therefore likely to seek help for their problems (Santhya et al. 2014). In addition to this sociocultural explanation, it is also important to review the gender differences through a developmental lens. A review of longitudinal studies has found that prevalence of specific disorders changes as children transition into adolescence and later into adulthood, and this was different for girls and boys (Costello et al. 2011). Substance use disorders, autism spectrum disorders and psychosis were found to be more common among adolescent boys, while depression and anxiety were more common among adolescent girls. The study found that as adolescents transition into adulthood, prevalence of substance use disorders, panic disorders and eating disorders continues to increase, while behavioural disorders, ADHD and specific phobias and generalised anxiety disorder tend to decrease.

Longitudinal studies on depression have found that prevalence of depression increases through adolescence and adulthood (Merikangas et al. 2009). While gender differences are not found in the age of onset of depression, studies have shown higher rates of depression among preadolescent boys but during adolescence rates are higher among females than males (Merikangas et al. 2009). In addition to common mental health disorders, body image concerns and eating disorders are also quite common among girls and young women. A study conducted with 120 females between the ages 13 and 17 years in Uttar Pradesh found that 26.67% of the participants experienced disturbed attitudes towards eating and showed presence of symptoms of eating disorders (Upadhyah et al. 2014). In another study of 586 adolescent girls between the ages 10 and 19 years from rural, slums and urban areas, 26.6% girls reported being completely dissatisfied with their bodies and 20.5% girls indicated a desire to become thin (Dixit et al. 2011).). Of the girls who were satisfied with their body image, 32.8% girls were underweight, and 38.4% were stunted (Dixit et al. 2011). While many studies document the high prevalence of body image issues among female adolescents, boys too experience similar concerns as reported in Basker et al. (2013) but there is limited documentation of the same. Given these findings and acknowledging that adolescence is a period of biological development and puberty, it is important to understand the role of gender in the context of the developmental trajectories of different psychological disorders. This will help identify the developmentally appropriate needs of boys and girls and design programmes and services to address the same.

In the studies reviewed, adolescent girls reported emotional problems more than boys (Reddy et al. 2011), while boys report higher peer-related problems than their female counterparts (Bhola et al. 2016). This is consistent with literature internationally which shows that young girls experience emotional problems like depression more than young men (Albert 2015; Priess et al. 2009). While this may be attributed to under-reporting by boys, this may also be linked to the process of gender socialisation and intensification. As young girls and boys enter adolescence, they get influenced by sociocultural roles and identities and begin to adopt the stereotypical gendered attitudes and identity roles. Boys begin to see themselves as being more "masculine" while girls being to imbibe the more "feminine traits" which can further influence their experience of depressive symptoms (Priess et al. 2009). In their attempt to understand the gender differences in depression, Preiss et al. (2009) have argued that stereotypical notions of masculinity are often associated with high self-efficacy, self-esteem and perceived competence which decreases the likelihood of depression, while femininity is often associated with sacrifice, high emotionality and helpless styles of coping with stressful situations which is likely to increase depressive symptoms. A study of depression among Canadian teenagers has supported this gender intensification hypothesis. The study found that older adolescent girls who adopted highly feminine role-related characteristics such as being responsible for others' welfare and not being assertive also reported higher depressive symptoms (Aubé et al. 2000). However, the literature on this is inconsistent and limited, but it offers great insight to explore the role of gender socialisation in adolescent mental health. Gender differences also play a role in the onset of depression with research reporting higher prevalence rates among adolescent girls because of hormonal changes and puberty (Albert 2015; Angold et al. 1999). In addition to hormonal markers, adolescent girls in India are at high risk for sexual abuse and violence accounting for 24% of rape cases in the country (National Crime Records Bureau 2012). As per the records of the National Crime Records Bureau (2012), over 8000 adolescent girls in India between the ages 10 and 18 years reported being raped. Child marriage is still prevalent in India with many young girls getting married before the age of 18 years (Raj et al. 2010; Speizer and Pearson 2010) and are therefore also more vulnerable to intimate partner violence (Speizer and Pearson 2010). The presence of such stressful life events place women at a higher risk for mental health concerns like depression and anxiety. It is important, therefore, to take into consideration the physiological and social aspects of vulnerability while understanding the role of gender in onset and maintenance of mental health concerns.

3.3.2.6 Prevalence of Psychological Disorders Across Urban and Rural Settings

Geographical location and socio-economic conditions also influence the reported prevalence of psychological disorders, as well as help-seeking behaviours. The Census (2011) data shows that prevalence of mental retardation is much higher among adolescents in rural India (0.02%) than among urban adolescents (0.009%). The data also reveals that while 72,225 rural Indian adolescents accounting for 0.005% of the total population are living with a mental illness, only 28,971 adolescents in urban India (0.002%) have a mental illness (Census 2011). This is, however, not congruent with recent data from the NIMHANS National Mental Health Survey which shows that prevalence of psychological disorders is nearly twice (13.5%) as much in urban metros as compared to rural (6.9%) areas among adolescents in the age group 13–17 years (NIMHANS 2016). Similar trends were found in a study of 2048 adolescents from urban and rural Goa where prevalence of psychological disorders among urban adolescents from English-speaking homes was higher (Pillai et al. 2008). While the NIMHANS survey only includes data from four states and the other study is limited to one state, it is important to acknowledge the factors that may have contributed to this incongruence in findings between these studies and the Census data. Firstly, the definition of mental illness was different across all studies. Secondly, while the Census relies on self-reported data, the other studies used clinically standardised screening tools. This may account for under-reporting in the Census data. Globally too, the literature on the relationship between geographical setting and mental illnesses among adolescents is not conclusive. In a comparative study of prevalence of mental illnesses and depression among adolescents in urban and rural areas in the USA, no statistically significant associations were found between the setting and prevalence rates among adolescents (Breslau et al. 2014).

While factors such as lifestyle, stress and academic pressures may be speculated as possible reasons for higher prevalence rates in urban areas among adolescents in India, further research is needed to support this argument.

3.3.2.7 Role of Socio-economic Factors in Prevalence of Psychological Disorders

Prevalence of psychological disorders has been found across all social classes (Gaur et al. 2003) but has not been extensively studied yet. Those belonging to the lower socio-economic classes could be at higher risk for psychological disorders (Rahi et al. 2005). Poor social and economic conditions bring with it many other problems like unsafe living conditions, difficulty accessing healthcare services, lack of education and awareness about mental health, etc. which have found to be associated with higher prevalence of psychological disorders among adolescents (Pillai et al. 2008). In addition to socio-economic class, the caste system is also a significant correlate in the Indian context. Certain castes and tribes are recognised by the Government of India as being economically and socially disadvantaged. While the importance of studying the role of caste in the context of prevalence of psychological disorders is recognised (Cheng et al. 2016), there is absence of conclusive literature on this.

Additionally, it is important to recognise that globalisation has an enormous impact on the culture and economy of developing nations. The gap between the rich and poor keeps increasing resulting in further marginalisation of certain sections of society. These sections of the population are therefore at a higher risk for mental health concerns. On the other hand, the urban population and upwardly mobile adolescents are exposed to many alternate cultures and come under pressure to keep up with the same. It is important, therefore to also explore and study the role and impact of changing cultural trends on adolescent mental health (Pillai et al. 2008).

3.3.2.8 Mental Health of School-Going Adolescents

The above review indicates the high prevalence of psychological disorders among the country's young population. It is important to recognise that much of this population is of school-going age. The role of the school and its significance in addressing adolescent mental health therefore becomes critical. Of the large young population in India, 63.02% adolescents between the ages 11 and 18 years are enrolled in primary and secondary schools (MHRD, Government of India 2011). School enrolment data from the Ministry of Human Resource Development also shows that the gross enrolment ratio ranges from 60 to 80% for upper primary (classes 6–8) and secondary and senior secondary (classes 9–12) levels of education. This indicates the need to identify the potential of young people in schools and create safe school environments that promote health and wellbeing of all students. The high prevalence rates of psychological disorders among adolescents reiterate the need for such initiatives.

As seen in Table 3.1, studies conducted in schools and colleges report high prevalence of emotional difficulties (Ahmad et al. 2007; Mishra and Sharma 2001; Chandrashekarappa et al. 2016) and behavioural concerns (Reddy et al. 2011; NIMHANS 2015; Bhola et al. 2016). In contrast, studies conducted with similar age groups in community settings do not report similarly high prevalence rates of emotional difficulties but report higher prevalence of disorders like enuresis, phobias and behavioural concerns (Srinath et al. 2005; Patil et al. 2013). It may be deliberated that schooling and education may play a role in the adolescents' ability to acknowledge their feelings and articulate their emotional distress resulting in higher reporting of emotional difficulties. On the other hand, it is also likely that school-going adolescents may experience different stressors like examination, academic pressures, peer conflicts, competition, etc. which may increase their vulnerability and risk for emotional and behavioural problems. While these are speculations without any supporting evidence, this finding highlights the significant role of schools in addressing emotional and mental health needs of adolescents. Similar recommendations for school-based mental health interventions have been documented nationally and internationally. The differences in prevalence rates in school-based studies and community settings have been documented earlier (Bhola and Kapur 2003) and are important from the perspective of designing setting-based interventions and services.

3.3.3 Risk and Protective Factors

Mental health of adolescents and youth is influenced by several factors. Some of these work as protective factors and can prevent the development of psychological disorders, while some act as risks and can accelerate or increase the likelihood of developing a psychological disorder. These risk and protective factors can be categorised into three domains: biological, psychological and social (WHO 2005). Ministry of Health and Family Welfare (2014) identifies various social factors such as homelessness, overcrowding, unsafe drinking water and sanitation, micronutrient deficiency, etc. as risk factors. The role of family and social support as protective factors and academic stressors as risk factors has been identified (Mehta et al. 2015). While these factors serve as mediators and not determinants, the role of protective factors in modifying and eliminating risk factors as well as mitigating the prevalence of risk behaviours has been identified (Patel and Goodman 2007).

Mental health of adolescents is also found to be influenced negatively if there is a family history of psychopathology (Srinath et al. 2005). In addition to genetic and biological factors, factors like family circumstances, large family sizes or nuclear families (Patil et al. 2013), parental discord, separation of parents or death of a parent, financial difficulties at home (Bhola et al. 2016), alcohol abuse in the father (Rahi et al. 2005), lack of father's interest in adolescent's life (Verma et al. 2001) and poor relationship with parents (Mishra and Sharma 2001) have been identified as risk factors. Experiences ranging from school-related academic difficulties

(Verma et al. 2001; Rahi et al. 2005) to physical abuse (Pillai et al. 2008) are found to increase the risk of developing psychological disorders.

Marital status of adolescent girls is also a significant factor that influences mental health. In the study of AFHCs across three states in India as discussed in Sect. 3.3.2 (Santhya et al. 2014), it was found that married young women reported psychological disorders much more (27.9%) as compared to unmarried young women (20.9%). This makes it important to explore the role of social responsibilities and possible risk factors like domestic violence that may be experienced by married women. The study found that the number of young women seeking help was highest in Maharashtra as compared to Jharkhand and Rajasthan. The study reported that Maharashtra is more urbanised and the awareness of mental health and healthcare services is more in this state than the other two states and the higher rates of help-seeking may be attributed to these factors (Santhya et al. 2014). The kind of risk and protective factors vary across the different sociocultural contexts within India. An in-depth understanding of the relationship between risk factors, protective factors and vulnerability among adolescents and youth is essential in developing programmes to strengthen protective factors and promote mental wellbeing.

3.3.4 Cross-Cutting Issues: Treatment Gap, Stigma and Discrimination, Social Vulnerabilities

In India, as discussed above, the prevalence of psychological disorders among adolescents and young people is high and in need of immediate attention. According to the NIMHANS survey, 9.8 million young people in the country are in need of specialised mental healthcare services (NIMHANS 2016). However, there is a dearth of mental health professionals in the country with only 3800 psychiatrists and 898 clinical psychologists in the country (Ministry of Health and Family Welfare 2017). This wide gap makes many services inaccessible to adolescents and young people.

In regions where services are available and accessible too, lack of awareness about mental health in the general population results in delayed identification (Mishra et al. 2011; Lahariya et al. 2010) and under reporting of mental health concerns. Further, the stigma associated with mental health results in neglect and marginalisation of those with a psychological disorder (NIMHANS 2016). The stigmatisation of psychological disorders across all age groups decreases the likelihood of individuals and families seeking assistance or mental healthcare services to avoid embarrassment and discrimination. During the consultative meet, while identifying stigma as a key barrier to help-seeking among adolescents, an expert noted, "Stigma is a big challenge. If mental hospitals were called positive health centres, more young people would access it".

Stigma and discrimination can be strong barriers towards seeking intervention, and this has to be taken into consideration during strategic planning for service programmes. In the study of AFHCs, it was found that only 31–33% of young women and men who reported psychological disorders sought advice and/or treatment for the same (Santhya et al. 2014). The study used detailed questionnaires to assess treatment seeking among adolescents and young people approaching the AFHCs. The major reasons cited by those who did not seek treatment were the perception that the mental health concern was not serious (84–94%), the feeling of embarrassment (3–10%) and the lack of money to seek treatment (4–16%). They also used qualitative methods of inquiry by conducting exit interviews with those who sought treatment and interviews with all health professionals including Auxiliary Nurse Midwives (ANMs) and counsellors at the AFHCs to assess help-seeking behaviour and the effectiveness of the services delivered. Data from these sources showed that there was hardly any awareness about AFHCs among young men and women (4.5% in young men and 7.8% in young women) despite their villages being located within 5–10 km from the clinics. This shows that it is important to create awareness about mental health among adolescents and youth to break the stigma and empower them to seek help. The role of stigma as a barrier to help-seeking behaviour has been established in mental health literature and was also recently recognised by the NIMHANS survey (2016). In a study of first year medical undergraduate students between the ages 17 and 19 years in South India, it was found that students have unfavourable attitudes towards seeking help from mental health professionals (Sameed et al. 2016). The study provided the respondents with a hypothetical case vignette of a student experiencing depression and found that 59.9% of the respondents did not feel the need for the subject in the case vignette to seek professional help. They reported that speaking to friends and family would suffice. Only 30.7% suggested seeking help from a counsellor, and only 11.7% reported the need to seek help from a psychiatrist. The researchers have deliberated that these results may be attributed to the stigma and negative attitudes associated with mental illness (Sameed et al. 2016). There are a range of studies which identify the need to reduce stigma to encourage help-seeking among adolescents in schools and colleges (Sodhi and Kakkar 2014; Kodad and Kazi 2014; Rajagopal 2013), and it is important therefore to acknowledge the same.

Adolescent mental health problems are often not given adequate significance, and parents of these individuals are often blamed and do not receive support from the community (WHO 2005), thereby highlighting the need to create adequate awareness about adolescent mental health and prevalence of psychological disorders in adolescence. The WHO Mental Health Service and Guideline Package (2005) also mentions that prevalent community beliefs around psychological disorders being caused due to spiritual factors often result in exclusion and isolation of individuals suffering from mental illness and comes in their way of seeking psychiatric help. In a study of 360 participants from urban and rural areas of Delhi ranging from 15 years to those above 56 years, it was found using a detailed questionnaire that 39.6% of the rural sample and 20.7% of the urban sample believed that mental disorders were “God’s punishment for past sins” (Kishore et al. 2011). The same study also included a separate sample of 76 medical professionals from Delhi, of which 5.2% believed mental disorders to be related to past sins. The study also found that individuals across various age groups and also respondents belonging to the medical profession held many myths and misconceptions about mental health, and this was more prevalent in rural areas. These beliefs are strongly rooted barriers in the process of addressing mental health needs of the young population in India.

In addition to stigma associated with mental health, many sociocultural circumstances and factors may place young individuals at higher risk for discrimination. One of the experts identified various vulnerable groups of adolescents and youth such as children of prisoners, children of women in sex work, homeless youth (particularly girls), children of homeless families, children in conflict with law and children in need for care and protection who require immediate attention and targeted action. While some studies on children in conflict with law identify adolescents as a vulnerable group (Mehta 2008; Malhotra et al. 2007), they are limited to including adolescents below the age of 18 years. It is important therefore to study the heterogeneity in this group and identify the specific needs of adolescents in vulnerable circumstances.

Another expert mentioned that young individuals in disaster-affected areas show high prevalence of disorders like post-traumatic stress disorder (PTSD), acute stress disorder and depression as responses to the stress, and their needs often stretch beyond treatment with a larger focus on rehabilitation. Experts also reported that adolescents and youth in conflict areas like Kashmir and areas affected by Naxalite-Maoist insurgency also seem to show a high prevalence of psychological disorders like anxiety disorders, panic attacks, depression, social phobia and somatisation and therefore require specialised interventions and services. In a study of 2728 individuals including school-going adolescents above the age of 16 years and college-going youth from various rural and urban districts of Kashmir, prevalence of depression was found to be highest (66.67%) in the age group 15–25 years and was higher for females than males (Amin and Khan 2009). A study of mental health of 150 adolescents and youth between the ages 15 and 25 years in Kashmir, using the State-Trait Anxiety Inventory (STAI) and the WHO Self-Reporting Questionnaire-20, found that respondents who had faced a violent episode scored higher on neuroticism; were more likely to experience phobias, psychosomatic symptoms, suspiciousness, fatigue, tension; and had lower frustration tolerance (Mir et al. 2016). Identifying and addressing the impact of political violence on mental health of adolescents and youth is therefore important and critical.

Sexual abuse was another area identified as requiring immediate action. One of the experts pointed out that some adolescents may not identify physical and sexual abuse especially when it is non-contact abuse like watching porn. Boys may also fear reporting the same because of social expectations of being brave and courageous. In addition to the above-mentioned groups, adolescents and young people from marginalised backgrounds, particularly those belonging to the tribal population and those expressing alternate sexualities, were identified as being especially vulnerable to psychological disorders, during the consultative meet, and as key vulnerable groups requiring serious urgent attention.

As seen through the data above, adolescent and youth in India, across different socio-economic classes, gender and geographical regions, are experiencing psychological disorders. The *Mental Health Policy and Service Guidance Package* (WHO 2005) identifies three significant reasons for establishing mental health services and interventions for children and adolescents. First, these services will allow early identification of mental health problems as disorders will be recognised at the onset. Second, many psychological disorders that begin to present during adolescence and youth may continue into adulthood and lead to impairment and disability. Therefore, adolescent mental health requires immediate and urgent attention to prevent onset of lifelong mental illnesses. Third, these interventions can help reduce the impact and burden of mental illness on the individual, family, society and nation. Establishing mental health service plans for adolescents and youth is a large-scale process and does not come under the purview of this chapter. However, the chapter attempts to identify possible course of action and recommendations for future research and programmatic implementation for adolescent and youth mental health promotion and advocacy, prevention and intervention.

3.4 Recommendations for Future Course of Action

Based on the review of epidemiological data and inputs from the interviews and consultations, the burden of mental illness, as well as the immediate need to address psychological disorders of adolescents and youth in India, is strongly evident. In view of this understanding, this chapter presents three priority areas of action to address the mental health needs of adolescents and youth in the country. Table 3.3 presents key strategies in the context of the priority areas of action.

Table 3.3 Areas of action and strategic recommendations to address adolescent and youth mental health needs in India

Sr. No.	Area of action	Strategies
1.	*Research*	Establish a research hub
		Study the role of social factors
		Study needs and challenges of adolescents and youth
2.	*Service design and delivery*	Review existing programmes and initiatives
		Optimising potential of schools and colleges as mental health sites
		Develop community programmes and train community workers
		Strengthen and initiate contextually relevant suicide prevention programmes
3.	*Advocacy*	Design programmes to promote adolescent and youth mental health across various settings including virtual platforms
		Develop campaigns and other initiatives to generate awareness, reduce stigma and encourage help-seeking for mental health needs

3.4.1 Research

The existing research on adolescent and youth mental health is scattered across clinical studies conducted in healthcare centres and hospitals and community-based studies conducted in schools or community settings. Due to this there has been limited national-level data. Further, the heterogeneity of this group makes it difficult to generalise the findings of existing research. It is therefore essential to develop a common repository of research on adolescents and youth across various setting sand contexts in India.

3.4.1.1 Establish a Research Hub

In India, the differences in cultures and socio-political environments from one region to another make it imperative to take these factors into consideration while studying health and mental health in those regions. This reiterates the need for research across all states and regions to identify contextually specific needs and challenges. However, it is equally essential to gather such diverse data and review it critically to identify common trends and needs of adolescents in the country. It is important to develop a dedicated task force that reviews existing research, identifies the gaps and limitations and proposes new research studies to address the existing challenges. This task force can also engage in qualitative research to bring forth narratives of adolescents and youth experiencing emotional distress and those seeking psychological help. Initiating research on hitherto less researched topics like pathological gambling, Internet addiction, eating disorders and compulsive sexual behaviours among adolescents in urban and rural areas is also essential. Such efforts will create a comprehensive understanding of adolescent- and youth-specific mental health needs in India.

3.4.1.2 Study the Role of Social Factors

Given the significant role played by various sociocultural factors in influencing the onset and course of various psychological disorders as discussed in Sect. 3.3.3, it is important to study the relationship between these factors and the psychological disorders. To begin this process, it is important to acknowledge that some risk and protective factors are contextually driven, and it is essential to assess these using relevant tools and methods. As discussed in Sect. 3.3.2, most epidemiological studies use screening tools based on clinical symptoms identified by diagnostic manuals like the *Diagnostic and Statistical Manual* or *International Classification of Diseases*. These checklists do not always account for sociocultural variations specific to different communities and cultures. It is important therefore to develop contextually relevant standardised screening tools that assess for protective and risk factors that influence the mental health of adolescents and youth in the country.

3.4.1.3 Study Needs and Challenges of Adolescents and Youth

This chapter highlights the heterogeneity of the group of adolescents and youth and the need to conduct more studies to identify the mental health needs of vulnerable populations within this group. As discussed in Sect. 3.3.3, the risk factors experienced by vulnerable groups of adolescents have not been studied in the Indian context. Including the mental health needs of adolescents and youth in conflict with law, transgender adolescents and youth, HIV-positive young individuals and young people experiencing marginalisation is important and significant to the discourse on adolescent and youth mental health.

3.4.2 Service Design and Delivery

The need for services and programmes to address adolescent- and youth-specific needs has been identified in the introduction of the chapter. It is important to design these programmes and services to effectively meet the needs of this group across various contexts across all levels of care including promotion, prevention and intervention.

3.4.2.1 Review Existing Programmes and Initiatives

The status of adolescent and youth mental health is concerning and in need of immediate intervention. However, there are many programmes and services that are already contributing to address these challenges and enhance adolescent and youth mental health. It is important therefore to review them, identify their scope, assess the impact and explore the possibilities of strengthening these initiatives and expanding these programmes.

3.4.2.2 Optimise Potential of Schools and Colleges as Mental Health Sites

Considering that a sizeable proportion of adolescents are enrolled in and attend school and could be experiencing academic, social and developmental stressors, it is important therefore to ensure that schools, colleges and universities are safe spaces for them. Academic institutions could emerge as effective platforms for discussions on mental health awareness and can further develop programmes and interventions to address needs of those at risk for psychological disorders. It will be equally essential to identify the challenges that these settings pose and ways to mobilise existing resources to meet these challenges.

3.4.2.3 Develop Community Programmes and Train Community Workers

The treatment gap in mental health has been acknowledged since years and also identified as a significant challenge in this chapter. This makes it essential to train healthcare providers and community workers in early identification, screening and referral for adolescent- and youth-specific psychological disorders. It is also important to review any such ongoing practices in India and internationally and to adapt and strengthen these models at the national level.

3.4.2.4 Strengthen and Initiate Contextually Relevant Suicide Prevention Programmes

As discussed in Sect. 3.3.2, suicide is a significant mental health concern for the young population. In order to develop effective strategies to prevent adolescent suicides, existing services like crisis helplines, prevention and intervention projects need to be reviewed to assess their effectiveness and impact. At the same time, reviewing international programmes that have been impactful will also be useful in designing new programmes. It is important to create action plans and programmes in healthcare settings, schools and colleges to generate awareness about warning signs of suicide and train first-line respondents in these settings like teachers and medical officers and also parents and peers in how to provide support to children and adolescents at risk for self-harm or suicide.

3.4.3 Advocacy

Adolescent and youth mental health has not received the kind of attention it needs within the community, and the myths and misconceptions associated with it continue to remain. It is essential therefore to create awareness about the mental health needs of adolescents and youth and strive to reduce the stigma associated with it.

3.4.3.1 Design Programmes to Promote Adolescent and Youth Mental Health Across Various Settings Including Virtual Platforms

Promoting adolescent mental health requires involvement of various stakeholders including mental health professionals, school and college authorities, healthcare providers, policy-makers and community organisations. Developing campaigns to highlight the role of mental health in overall wellbeing is significant in encouraging the community to address mental health needs seriously. As discussed in Sect. 3.3.2, the number of adolescents and young individuals using the Internet is increasing. It is essential therefore to utilise virtual platforms such as the *youthinfoindia* youth portal, social media and other blogs to reach out to young individuals and empower them.

3.4.3.2 Develop Campaigns and Other Initiatives to Generate Awareness, Reduce Stigma and Encourage Help-Seeking for Mental Health Needs

In order to encourage adolescents and young people to seek help and respond to their mental health needs, it is important to address the existing misconceptions about mental health within the community. This can be done through various community initiatives or awareness drives. Developing online content and Information, Education and Communication (IEC) resources in local languages is also a great way to generate awareness about adolescent and youth needs. Initiating public discussions in common spaces like clubs, schools and community grounds during health camps is also a good way to destigmatise mental health and make it part of the public health discourse.

3.5 Conclusion

The mental health and wellbeing of adolescents and youth are extremely important to ensure a productive task force and an illness-free and healthy generation of future adults. While adolescents and youth are at high risk for various psychological disorders, it is important to address these risk factors through concerted efforts and interventions in various settings. It is equally important to identify the strengths and protective factors that the adolescents and the environment possess and their role in promoting mental health. The potential of adolescents in preventing psychological disorders and enhancing their own wellbeing is critical to this dialogue. Factors like resilience and social capacities can play a major role in shifting the lens from problem-focused resolutions to strength-based discussions generating opportunities and hope for change. This chapter provides an overview of adolescent and youth mental health needs and the possible course of action for mental health professionals, academicians and programme developers. However, it is important to complement this data with reviews of existing systems and processes to address these needs in the country. An extensive review of the existing policies and programmes addressing adolescent and youth mental health needs in the country will provide a more comprehensive picture of the adolescent and youth mental health status in India.

Acknowledgements We would like to thank all the officials from the Ministry of Health and Family Welfare, Government of India; representatives from the State Government of Maharashtra; representatives from the RKSK programme; policy-makers and experts who participated in the consultative meet; experts from the National Institute of Mental Health and Neurosciences (NIMHANS), Bengaluru; practicing mental health professionals; and faculty at the Tata Institute of Social Sciences, Mumbai, for their invaluable inputs and recommendations.

References

Ahmad, A., Khalique, N., Khan, Z., & Amir, A. (2007). Prevalence of psychosocial problems among school going male adolescents. *Indian Journal of Community Medicine, 32*(3), 219–221.

Albert, P. R. (2015, July). Why is depression more prevalent in women? *Journal of Psychiatry and Neuroscience, 40*(4), 219–221. https://doi.org/10.1503/jpn.150205.

Amin, S., & Khan, A. W. (2009). Life in conflict: Characteristics of depression in Kashmir. *International Journal of Health Sciences, 3*(2), 213–223.

Angold, A., Costello, E. J., & Worthman, C. W. (1999). Puberty and depression: The roles of age, pubertal status, and pubertal timing. *Psychological Medicine, 28*, 51–61.

Arun, P., & Chavan, B. (2009). Stress and suicidal ideas in adolescent students in Chandigarh. *Indian Journal of Medical Sciences, 63*(7), 281–287.

Aubé, J., Fichman, L., Saltaris, C., & Koestner, R. (2000). Gender differences in adolescent depressive symptomatology: Towards an integrated social-developmental model. *Journal of Social and Clinical Psychology, 19*(3), 297–313. https://doi.org/10.1521/jscp.2000.19.3.297.

Basker, M., Mathai, S., Korula, S., & Mammen, P. M. (2013). Eating disorders among adolescents in a tertiary Care Centre in India. *Indian Journal of Pediatrics, 80*(3), 211–214. Retrieved from https://link.springer.com/article/10.1007/s12098-012-0819-4.

Belfer, M. L. (2005). Child and adolescent mental health around the World: Challenges for progress. *Journal of Indian Association for Child and Adolescent Mental Health, 1*(1).

Bhola, P., & Kapur, M. (2003). Child and adolescent psychiatric epidemiology in India. *Indian Journal of Psychiatry, 45*, 208–217.

Bhola, P., Sathyanarayanan, V., Rekha, D. P., Daniel, S., & Thomas, T. (2016). Assessment of self-reported emotional and behavioral difficulties among pre-university college students in Bangalore, India. *Indian Journal of Community Medicine, 41*(2), 146–150.

Breslau, J., Marshall, G. N., Pincus, H. A., & Brown, R. A. (2014). Are mental disorders more common in urban than rural areas of the United States? *Journal of Psychiatric Research*. https://doi.org/10.1016/j.jpsychires.2014.05.004.

Chandrasekhar, C. P., Ghosh, J., & Rowchowdhury, A. (2006, January). The 'Demographic Dividend' and young India's economic future. *Economic and Political Weekly, 41*(49), 5055–5064.

Chandrashekarappa, S. M., Ramakrishnaiah, N. M., Ram, D., & Manjunath, R. (2016). Mental Helath among adolescent girls – An effort to know the association of mental disorders with socio-demographic variables. *International Journal of Medical Science and Public Health, 5*(11).

Cheng, H. G., Shidhaye, R., Charlson, F., Deng, F., Lyngdoh, T., Chen, S., et al. (2016). Social correlates of mental, neurological, and substance use disorders in China and India: A review. *The Lancet Psychiatry, 3*(9), 882–899. https://doi.org/10.1016/S2215-0366(16)30166-3.

Costello, E. J., Copeland, W., & Angold, A. (2011). Trends in psychopathology across the adolescent years: What changes when children become adolescents, and when adolescents become adults? *Journal of Child Psychology and Psychiatry, 52*(10), 1015–1025. https://doi.org/10.1111/j.1469-7610.2011.02446.x.

Dixit, S., Agarwal, G. G., Singh, J. V., Kant, S., & Singh, N. (2011). A study on consciousness of adolescent girls about their body image. *Indian Journal of Community Medicine, 36*(3), 197–202. https://doi.org/10.4103/0970-0218.86520.

Gaur, A. D., Vohra, A., Subash, S., & Khurana, H. (2003). Prevalence of psychiatric morbidity among 6 to 14 years old chldren. *Indian Journal of Community Medicine, 28*(3), 133–137.

Goel, D., Subramanyam, A., & Kamath, R. (2013). A study on the prevalence of internet addiction and its association with psychopathology in Indian adolescents. *Indian Journal of Psychiatry, 55*(2), 140–143. https://doi.org/10.4103/0019-5545.111451.

Government of India Ministry of Human Resource Development. (2011). *Educational statistics at a glance*. New Delhi: Government of India Ministry of Human Resource Development. Retrieved from https://mhrd.gov.in/sites/upload_files/mhrd/files/statistics-new/EduStatGlance_2011_0.pdf.

Gururaj, G., Pradeep, B. S., Beri, G., Chauhan, A., & Rizvi, Z. (2014). *Adolescent and youth health survey- Himachal Pradesh 2014*. Bangalore: Centre for Public Health, National Institute of Mental Health and NeuroSciences.

Hindustan Times. (2017, May 30). Suicide city' Kota's new preventive tactic is ceiling fans with springs, sirens. *Hindustan Times*.

Jaisoorya, T. S., Beena, K. V., Beena, M., Jose, D. C., Ellangovan, K., Thennarasu, K., & Benegal, V. (2016). Prevalence & correlates of tobacco use among adolescents in Kerala, India. *Indian Journal of Medical Research, 144*(5), 704–711. Retrieved from https://www.ncbi.nlm.nih.gov/pmc/articles/PMC5393081/.

Jhala, J., & Sharma, R. (2017). Prevalence and nature of internet use among adolescents in Vadodara (Gujarat). *The International Journal of Indian Psychology, 4*(2), 28–42.

Jones, P. B. (2013). Adult mental health disorders and their age at onset. *The British Journal of Psychiatry.* https://doi.org/10.1192/bjp.bp.112.119164.

Kelleher, I., Connor, D., Clarke, M. C., Devlin, N., Harley, M., & Cannon, M. (2012). Prevalence of psychotic symptoms in childhood and adolescence: A systematic review and meta-analysis of population-based studies. *Psychological Medicine, 42*(9), 1857–1863. https://doi.org/10.1017/S0033291711002960.

Kishore, J., Gupta, A., Jiloha, R. C., & Bantman, P. (2011). Myths, beliefs and perceptions about mental disorders and health-seeking behavior in Delhi, India. *Indian Journal of Psychiatry, 53*(4), 324–329. https://doi.org/10.4103/0019-5545.91906.

Kleinert, S., & Horton, R. (2016). Adolescent health and wellbeing: A key to a sustainable future. *The Lancet, 387*(10036), 2355–2356.

Kodad, H. S., & Kazi, S. A. (2014). Emerging area of counselling in schools in India. *International Research Journal of Social Sciences, 3*(3), 44–47.

Lakhan, R., & Ekúndayò, O. T. (2015, Jan–Mar). National sample survey organization survey report: An estimation of prevalence of mental illness and its association with age in India. *Journal of Neurosciences in Rural Practice, 6*(1), 51–54.

Lahariya, C., Singhal, S., Gupta, S., & Mishra, A. (2010). Pathway of care among psychiatric patients attending a mental health institution in Central India. *Indian Journal of Psychiatry, 52*(4), 333–338. https://doi.org/10.4103/0019-5545.74308.

Malhotra, S., & Patra, B. N. (2014). Prevalence of child and adolescent psychiatric disorders in India: A systematic review and meta-analysis. *Child and Adolescent Psychiatry and Mental Health, 8*(22).

Malhotra, C., Sharma, N., Saxena, R., & Ingle, G. (2007). Drug use among Juveniles in conflict with the law. *Indian Journal of Pediatrics, 74*, 35–38.

Math, S. B., & Srinivasaraju, R. (2010). Indian psychiatric epidemiological studies: Learning from the past. *Indian Journal of Psychiatry, 52*(7), 95–103.

Math, S. B., Chandrashekar, C. R., & Bhugra, D. (2007). Psychiatric epidemiology in India. *Indian Journal of Medical Research*, 183–192.

Mehta, N. (2008). *Child protection and juvenile justice system for children in need of care and protection*. Childline India Foundation. Retrieved from http://childlineindia.org.in/pdf/CP-JJ-CNCP.pdf.

Mehta, M., Pattanayak, R., & Sagar, R. (2015). Adolescent psychiatry: An overview of the Indian research. In S. Malhotra & S. Chakrabarti (Eds.), *Developments in psychiatry in India* (pp. 313–341). New Delhi: Springer India.

Merikangas, K. R., Nakamura, E. F., & Kessler, R. C. (2009). Epidemiology of mental disorders in children and adolescents. *Dialogues in Clinical Neuroscience, 11*(1), 7–20.

Ministry of Health and Family Welfare, Government of India. (2014, October). New pathways new Hope: National Mental Health Policy of India.

Ministry of Health and Family Welfare. (2017). Lok Sabha Unstarred Question No. 2709 - Shortge of Mental Healthcare Professionals. Government of India Ministry of Health and Family Welfare.

Mir, Z. S., Rather, Y. H., & Prusty, B. (2016). Effect of armed conflict on the mental health of youth in Kashmir. *International Journal of Contemporary Medical Research, 3*(5), 1409–1414.

Mishra, A., & Sharma, A. (2001). A clinico-social study of psychiatric morbidity in 12 to 18 years school going girls in urban Delhi. *Indian Journal of Community Medicine, 26*, 2.

Mishra, N., Nagpal, S. S., Chadda, R. K., & Sood, M. (2011). Help-seeking behavior of patients with mental health problems visiting a tertiary care center in North India. *Indian Journal of Psychiatry, 53*(3), 234–238. https://doi.org/10.4103/0019-5545.86814.

National Crime Records Bureau. (2012). *Crime in India 2012 statistics*. New Delhi: National Crime Records Bureau Ministry of Home Affairs. Retrieved from http://ncrb.gov.in/StatPublications/CII/CII2012/Statistics2012.pdf.

National Crime Records Bureau Ministry of Home Affairs. (2012). *Accidental deaths and suicides in India 2012*. New Delhi: National Crime Records Bureau Ministry of Home Affairs Government of India.

National Sample Survey Organisation, Ministry of Statistics and Programme Implementation, Government of India. (2002). *NSS 58th round (July - December 2002)*. Government of India.

NIMHANS. (2015). *Community Child & Adolescent Mental Health Service Project 2nd quarterly report, January to March 2015*. Dept. of Child & Adolescent Psychiatry, NIMHANS Supported by Dept. of Women & Child Development, Government of Karnataka. Retrieved from http://www.nimhanschildproject.in/reports/.

NIMHANS. (2016). *National Mental Health Survey of India 2015–16*. Bengaluru: National Institute of Mental Health and Neurosciences.

Nowinski, J. (1990). *Substance abuse in adolescents and young adults*. New York: Norton.

Office of the Registrar General and Census Commissioner, Ministry of Home Affairs, Government of India. (2011). *Census of India*. Retrieved August 2016, from population enumeration data (Final population): http://www.censusindia.gov.in/2011census/population_enumeration.html

Patel, V., & Goodman, A. (2007). Researching protective and promotive factors in mental health. *International Journal of Epidemiology, 36*(4), 703–707.

Patil, R. N., Nagaonkar, S. N., Shah, N. B., & Bhat, T. S. (2013). A Cross-sectional study of common psychiatric morbidity in children aged 5-14 years in an urban slum. *Journal of Family Medicine and Primary Care*, 165–168.

Pillai, A., Patel, V., Cardozo, P., Goodman, R., Weiss, H. A., & Andrew, G. (2008). Non-traditional lifestyles and prevalence of mental disorders in adolescents in Goa, India. *The British Journal of Psychiatry, 192*, 45–51.

Priess, H. A., Lindberg, S. M., & Hyde, J. S. (2009). Adolescent gender-role identity and mental health: Gender intensification revisited. *Child Development, 80*(5), 1531–1544. https://doi.org/10.1111/j.1467-8624.2009.01349.x.

Rahi, M., Kumavat, A., Garg, S., & Singh, M. (2005). Socio-demographic co-relates of psychiatric disorders. *Indian Journal of Pediatrics, 72*, 395–398.

Raj, A., Saggurti, N., Lawrence, D., Balaiah, D., & Silverman, J. G. (2010). Association between adolescent marriage and marital violence among young adult women in India. *International Journal of Gynecology & Obstetrics, 110*(1), 35–39. https://doi.org/10.1016/j.ijgo.2010.01.022.

Rajagopal, M. (2013). Counseling: A misunderstood profession. *IOSR Journal Of Humanities And Social Science (IOSR-JHSS), 11*(3), 30–37.

Reddy, B. K., Biswas, A., & Rao, H. (2011). Assessment of mental health of Indian adolescents studying in urban schools. *Malaysian Journal of Paediatrics and Child Health Online Early*.

Samanta, A., Mukherjee, S., Ghosh, S., & Dasgupta, A. (2012). Mental health, protective factors and violence among male adolescents: A comparison between urban and rural school students in West Bengal. *Indian Journal of Public Health, 56*(2), 155–158.

Sameed, S., Karkal, R., Mendonsa, R., Shriyan, S., Thomas, A. M., & Chandran, V. M. (2016, March). Help-seeking attitudes for depression among first year medical undergraduates. *Indian Journal of Basic and Applied Medical Research, 5*(2), 839–844.

Santhya, K. G., Prakash, R., Jejeebhoy, S. J., & Singh, S. (2014). *Accessing aolescent friendly health clinics in India: The perspectives of adolescents and youth*. New Delhi: Population Council.

Sharma, M., & Chaudhary, M. (2016). A study of drugs and substance abuse among adolescents of slum dwellers. *The International Journal of Indian Psychology, 4*(3), 20–27.

Singh, S., & Gururaj, G. (2014). Health behaviours & problems among young people in India: Cause for concern & call for action. *Indian Journal of Medical Research, 140*, 185–208.

Sinha, D. N. (2006). *Tobacco control in schools in India-India Global Youth Tobacco Survey & Global School Personnel Survey*. Ministry of Health and Family Welfare, Government of India.

Sodhi, K., & Kakkar, S. (2014). Youth and counselling in India- A study of the awareness levels and attitude of female urban college students towards professional counselling, and the effect of avoidance factors on help-seeking behaviour. *International Journal of Public Mental Health and Neurosciences, 1*(1), 23–33.

Speizer, I. S., & Pearson, E. (2010). Association between early marriage and intimate partner violence in India: A focus on youth from Bihar and Rajasthan. *Journal of Interpersonal Violence, 26*(10), 1963–1981. https://doi.org/10.1177/0886260510372947.

Srinath, S., Girimaji, S. C., Gururaj, G., Seshadri, S., Subbakrishna, D., Bhola, P., & Kumar, N. (2005, July). Epidemiological study of child & adolescent psychiatric disorders in urban and rural areas of Bangalore, India. *Indian Journal of Medical Research, 122*, 67–79.

Srivastava, S., Sharma, I., & Bhatia, M. S. (2014). Parenting in children and adolescents with psychosis. *Indian Pediatrics, 51*, 991–995.

Stevens, J. R., Prince, J. B., Prager, L. M., & Stern, T. A. (2014). Psychotic disorders in children and adolescents: A primer on contemporary evaluation and management. *The Primary Care Companion for CNS disorders, 16*(2). https://doi.org/10.4088/PCC.13f01514.

The Lancet. (2016). *Our future: A lancet commission on adolescent health and wellbeing*. The Lancet.

United Nations Children's Fund (UNICEF). (2011). *The State of the World's children: Adolescence an age of opportunity*. UNICEF.

United Nations Development Programme. (2014, August 12). *United Nations Development Programme (UNDP)*. Retrieved September 2016, from UN Secretary-General's Message on International Youth Day: http://www.in.undp.org/content/india/en/home/presscenter/pressreleases/2014/08/12/youthday2014.html

United Nations Population Fund (UNFPA). (2013). *UNFPA strategy on adolescents and youth*. New York: UNFPA.

Upadhyah, A., Misra, R., Parchwani, D., & Maheria, P. (2014). Prevalence and risk factors for eating disorders in Indian adolescent females. *National Journal of Physiology, Pharmacy & Pharmacology, 4*(2), 153–157.

Verma, M., Singh, T., Gupta, I., & Gupta, V. (2001). Behavioral problems in school-going children: Implications for medical teachers in developing countries. *Education for Health, 14*(2), 309–311.

Wallace, P. (2014). Internet addiction disorder and youth. *EMBO Reports, 15*(1), 12–16. https://doi.org/10.1002/embr.201338222.

World Health Organization (WHO). (2005). *Mental health policy and service guidance package: Child and adolescent mental health policies and plans*. Geneva: World Health Organization.

World Health Organization. (2014). *Preventing suicide: A global imperative*. World Health Organization.

World Health Organization. (2016). *Maternal, newborn, child and adolescent health*. Retrieved September 2016, from World Health Organization: http://www.who.int/maternal_child_adolescent/topics/adolescence/dev/en/

World Health Organization Department of Mental Health and Substance Dependence. (n.d.). *Gender disparities in mental health*.

Chapter 4
Adolescent and Youth Mental Health in India: Policies and Programmes

Chetna Duggal and Lamia Bagasrawala

Abstract India is set to become the youngest nation of the world with the largest youth population. It is important to nurture the young population and ensure their physical and mental health, so they can maximise their potential. However, the data on prevalence of psychological disorders among adolescents and young individuals indicates that a significant section of adolescents and youth is experiencing psychological disorders and psychosocial distress. It is important to address this and strengthen efforts at the national level towards enhancing adolescent and youth wellbeing. This chapter therefore aims to provide comprehensive information about existing policies related to adolescent and youth mental health and exploring the possibility of creating a new policy specific to this group. The chapter also reviews some selected programmes and initiatives developed in the country and attempts to weave them in the context of existing policies. The chapter concludes by proposing recommendations across various levels in the service delivery sector including research, policy and programme implementation to effectively address adolescent and youth needs in the country. The chapter is targeted at mental health professionals, researchers, adolescent and youth leaders, policy-makers and community organisations across the nation, with an aim to collaborate and create efficient and effective practices to enhance the mental health of adolescents and youth in India.

Keywords Adolescents and youth · Adolescent mental health · Youth mental health · Mental health policy · Mental health programmes

Adolescence and youth are significant periods of development and play a critical role in preparing an individual to live a psychologically, socially and economically fulfilling life as an adult. During adolescence and youth, individuals complete a vast array of developmental tasks which are aligned with their emotional, cognitive and

C. Duggal (✉)
School of Human Ecology, Tata Institute of Social Sciences, Mumbai, India
e-mail: chetna.d@tiss.edu

L. Bagasrawala
Tata Institute of Social Sciences, Mumbai, India

S. Bharat, G. Sethi (eds.), *Health and Wellbeing of India's Young People*,
https://doi.org/10.1007/978-981-13-6593-5_4

social growth. Physiological changes due to puberty, along with social responsibilities, relationships and other life stage-related demands such as examinations, can become challenging for many individuals as they navigate the adolescent years. While some individuals may cope well with the developmental challenges, others may experience distress and require support from friends and family; some others, however, may develop psychological concerns and require more professional support to help them transition into adulthood.

The estimates of prevalence of mental health problems among adolescents in the age group 10–19 years across different regions in India over the last 15 years have ranged from 0.20% (NSSO 2002) to 45.8% (Arun and Chavan 2009). In the recent National Mental Health Survey (2016) by the National Institute for Mental Health and Neurosciences (NIMHANS), the prevalence of psychological disorders among adolescents (13 to 17 years) across four states, using the Mini-International Neuropsychiatric Interview (MINI), was reported as 7.3%. Studies reveal that the most common mental health concerns experienced by adolescents are emotional difficulties such as anxiety and depression (Chandrashekarappa et al. 2016), neurodevelopmental concerns such as attention deficit hyperactivity disorder (ADHD) and behavioural concerns such as conduct disorder and oppositional defiant disorder (Pillai et al. 2008; Patil et al. 2013), substance use and psychosis (Gaur et al. 2003). Suicide is one of the leading mental health concerns among adolescents and youth requiring immediate attention (The Lancet 2016). Other psychosocial concerns such as peer problems (Reddy et al. 2011) and excessive use of the Internet (Goel et al. 2013) are also common among adolescents.

While mental health concerns are experienced by individuals across all social contexts, factors such as socio-economic conditions, socio-political situations, gender and geographic location may influence the onset, nature and course of a mental health problem experienced by an adolescent. Addressing the risks and strengthening the protective factors could help enhance adolescent mental health and reduce the prevalence of adolescent mental health concerns. Certain groups of adolescents and young people such as homeless youth, young individuals in conflict with law, adolescents living in conflict areas and areas affected by natural disasters and those from marginalised backgrounds are more vulnerable to psychological disorders than others. The existing data on adolescent mental health and their needs, discussed in the previous chapter, highlights the need to strengthen existing frameworks and programmes and design new services to prevent adolescent and youth mental health concerns and promote adolescent and youth wellbeing.

At the national level, policies are one of the most significant sources of guidelines that are developed to establish protocol. They provide a framework along which organisations and individuals can plan activities for the benefit of the country's citizens. Legal provisions and laws are other constitutionally upheld mandates for acceptable practices nationally. These legal documents and policies guide the designing and development of various programmes and services within the country. Since adolescent and youth mental health is an issue of national interest, it is important to understand and review the policies and legal documents that influence this discourse. While there is an absence of any one policy for adolescent and youth mental health in the country, it is critical to recognise how different policies address this issue within their purview. The impact of these policies is often assessed in the ways in which programmes operating in the country align with these policies. It is also crucial, therefore, to identify the best practices within the country, explore their strengths and explore the convergence between existing policies and programmes.

4.1 Methods

This chapter has been drafted after a detailed review of existing policies related to adolescent and youth mental health and selected programmes providing mental healthcare for adolescents and youth. Since there is no specific policy for adolescent and youth mental health, those policies were selected for review that included relevant mental health-related guidelines or guidelines for adolescents and youth. The Mental Health Care Act 2017 is the only law that has been included in this list. International provisions related to adolescent and youth mental health, which India as a country has signed to adhere to, have also been discussed. For the purpose of this chapter, all individuals between the ages 10 and 18 years are considered as adolescents and those between the ages 19 and 24 years as youth. The programmes reviewed have been selected based on expert recommendations or the significant work carried out by these organisations across specific areas of adolescent and youth mental health. The list of programmes reviewed is not exhaustive and is not representative of the national scenario. While the chapter highlights the best practices implemented by these organisations and programmes, it is not promoting them or disregarding the efforts of other programmes and interventions.

Reports published by various United Nations agencies as well as ministries of the Government of India have also been reviewed and cited whenever required, in addition to the policy and legal documents. The desk review and analysis were supplemented by expert views shared during the national consultative meet organised at the Tata Institute of Social Sciences (TISS), Mumbai campus, and information received from consultations with experts from the NIMHANS. The national consultative meet organised at TISS, Mumbai, focused on three broad areas of discussion related to mental health: status and future imperatives for national-level policies, programmatic level recommendations and exploration of possibilities for adolescent and youth engagement and leadership. The discussions and thoughts generated during this meet have been weaved into the chapter.

In Sect. 4.2, adolescent and youth mental health will be discussed in the context of various international and existing national-level policies. For ease of understanding, the national-level policies are presented in a tabular form along with key points related to adolescent and youth mental health. This is followed by a brief discussion on the need to develop an adolescent and youth mental health policy and the challenges related to it.

4.2 Adolescent and Youth Mental Health-Related Policies

Global- and national-level policies relevant to adolescent and youth mental health serve as guidelines to identify target groups and assess action areas for mental health interventions and services. During the consultations, experts emphasised the available potential of the existing policies in facilitating adolescent and youth mental health service development and the need for considerations for implementation at the centre and state level. This section of the chapter will identify global goals and mental health components related to adolescents and youth in different policies, as well as the gaps therein and its implications for adolescent and youth wellbeing.

4.2.1 At the Global Level: Locating Adolescents and Youth in MDGs and SDGs

India was one of the many nations to adopt the United Nation's Millennium Development Goals (MDGs) in the year 2000, with a purpose to bring about socio-economic development across various areas. While the MDGs focused on development in specific sectors to address issues of social and economic development, it did not explicitly identify mental health and wellbeing as an achievable goal. However, the role of mental health outcomes in facilitating achievement of the MDGs has been acknowledged. Psychological disorders like depression and anxiety, schizophrenia and drug abuse have been found to contribute significantly to the disability-affected life years (DALYs) and years lived with disability (YLDs) (Miranda and Patel 2005).

The MDGs which expired in 2015 were followed by the Sustainable Development Goals (SDGs), a list of 17 goals and 169 targets as part of the United Nations 2030 Agenda for Sustainable Development, seeking to continue the agenda of the MDGs. The SDGs identify the significance of mental health and wellbeing under Goal 3 which aims to ensure health and wellbeing for all individuals across all age groups which include adolescents and youth. It identifies the prevalence of mental disorders across different cultures with a special mention of depression- and anxiety-related disorders that may lead to suicide. Suicide has been recognised as a critical mental health concern requiring immediate attention under this goal. Although it identifies suicide as the second leading cause of death among adolescents and youth between the ages 15 and 29 years, there is no specific goal or mandate to address the mental health needs of this population within the SDG framework. Substance use and substance use disorders have also been identified as a major health concern under Goal 3 of the SDGs. The impact of alcohol consumption and drug use on public health has been acknowledged under this goal. In addition to specific mental health goals, the SDGs also recognise the role of mental wellbeing in achieving other developmental goals such as reducing mortality. However, the SDGs do not mention any specific outcome indicators or measurable parameters to assess the progress of the mental health-related goals in order to review the status of mental health and wellbeing.

In order to address this limitation, FundaMentalSDG, a global initiative led by mental health leaders in partnership with renowned mental health organisations from around the world, has proposed the inclusion of two indicators to assess mental health outcomes under the SDGs (FundaMentalSDG 2005). The proposed indicators are Indicator 23, probability of dying between ages 30 and 70 from any of cardiovascular disease, cancer, diabetes, chronic respiratory disease or suicide, and Indicator 28, proportion of persons with a severe mental disorder (psychosis, bipolar affective disorder or moderate-severe depression) who are using services. These indicators as suggested by the UN Sustainable Development Solutions Network (UNSDNS) are in line with the World Health Organization (WHO) Global Mental Health Action Plan 2013–2020 and aim to reduce the deaths caused by suicide and increase the service coverage for severe mental health disorders.

Despite the increasing burden of mental illness on economies around the world, mental health needs and outcomes have not received adequate prominence across the global development sector (Thornicroft and Votruba 2015), and there is an urgent need to integrate mental health outcomes within all relevant developmental programmes and frameworks.

4.2.2 Adolescent and Youth Mental Health in National Policies

Table 4.1 presents a brief overview of various national policies related to adolescent and youth mental health. For this chapter, the Mental Health Care Act 2017 has been included under the list of policies. Table 4.1 also highlights the key recommendations suggested by the policies for adolescent and youth mental health.

4.2.3 Need for an Adolescent and Youth Mental Health Policy

As seen in Table 4.1, the existing policies and legal guidelines offer a broad framework to initiate and plan actions to address mental health needs of adolescents and youth. Common adolescent mental health problems like depression, suicide and substance use have already been identified as key concerns requiring immediate action. The potential of schools and colleges and other youth spaces to address adolescent and youth mental health needs has also been recognised in these policies. The Mental Health Care Act 2017 (Government of India 2017) offers comprehensive mandates and guidelines for mental health services and the rights of adults and minors seeking mental healthcare in the country. Experts during the consultative meet recognised the National Mental Health Policy 2014 as a good set of comprehensive guidelines and recommended initiating action plans and programmes based on these directives. While all these policies identify the significance of adolescent and youth mental health in some way, there is absence of any single document focusing only on adolescent and youth mental health.

Table 4.1 Adolescent and youth mental health in national policies

Sr. No.	Name	Target population	Aim	Launched by	Recommendations for adolescent and youth wellbeing	Key points
1	*National Mental Health Policy 2014*	All individuals	To provide guidelines for mental health services and to approach mental health from a wellness perspective	Ministry of Health and Family Welfare, Govt. of India	1. Training teachers to provide Life Skills Education (LSE), addressing adolescents' distress and promoting mental health within schools	1. Shifts lens from an only treatment-oriented approach to a holistic approach including promotion, prevention, treatment and rehabilitation of those with psychological disorders
					2. Implementing LSE programmes in schools and colleges	2. Distinguishes between mental illness and mental health problems
					3. Providing young individuals with age- and context-specific knowledge through trained professionals	3. Identifies psychosocial distress and nonclinical disorders as valid mental health concerns requiring attention
					4. Setting up spaces like youth clubs to provide LSE skills to individuals who are not enrolled in schools and colleges	4. Acknowledges needs of vulnerable groups and other marginalised groups
					5. Early identification and intervention for mental disorders	5. Identifies adolescence as a critical period marking the onset of many mental health disorders like schizophrenia and mood disorders

2	*Mental Health Care Act 2017* Passed by the Parliament in the Lok Sabha in March 2017, and the Mental Health Act 1987 was repealed	All individuals		Ministry of Law and Justice, Govt. of India	1. Sub-clause *(e)* of sub-section *(4)* of clause 18 in Chapter V 'Rights of Persons with Mental Illness' of the Act identifies the rights of children to access mental health services without any prejudice 2. Identifies the need for easily accessible, good quality mental health services for *all* individuals with a special mention of district level services	1. Identifies specific needs of children and vulnerable groups such as children in orphanages, institutional care and children homes This implies that adolescents who are out-of-school or in institutional care are also entitled to mental health services 2. Decriminalisation of suicide is a mandate under this Act. Suicide is a major mental health concern among adolescents and youth. The Act identifies suicide as a stress-related mental health concern, attempts to destigmatise it and encourages individuals to seek help for the same

(continued)

Table 4.1 (continued)

Sr. No.	Name	Target population	Aim	Launched by	Recommendations for adolescent and youth wellbeing	Key points
3	*National Policy for Children 2013*	Children and individuals below the age of 18 years	To secure child rights and provide children with a safe, happy and healthy childhood	Ministry of Women and Child Development, Govt. of India	1. Initiating action to prevent mental disabilities among children and to prevent discrimination faced by children with disabilities	1. Identifies health as a priority area and recognises the need for comprehensive healthcare at promotive, preventive and rehabilitative levels
					2. Providing supportive and rehabilitative services for children at risk	2. Identifies need for holistic development of children across mental, emotional, cognitive, social and cultural domains
					3. Providing adolescents with information and support related to lifestyle choices, especially ill effects of alcohol and substance use	3. Acknowledges needs of vulnerable groups of children including street children, children with disabilities and children who use substances
					4. Holds the State responsible for protection of children from all forms of violence and abuse including sexual exploitation, pornography and substance use	4. Identifies adolescents as a target group in need of accurate information, adequate support and services to enhance their health and development
						5. To be reviewed every 5 years

4	*National Youth Policy 2014*	Youth in the age group 15–29 years	To identify key action areas for youth development and engagement	Ministry of Youth Affairs and Sports, Govt. of India	1. Initiating outreach programmes for youth engagement and collaboration with non-governmental organisations (NGOs) and private sector 2. Each State must create its own Youth Policy to address the sociocultural needs and concerns specific to youth in that given context	1. Priority area 4 recognises emotional and psychological disorders as a youth-specific issue requiring a targeted approach 2. Identifies the risk of depression and suicides among young people as well as the impact of substance use and the need to address them 3. Priority area 10 identifies need for inclusion of youth living in conflict-affected areas, those stigmatised because of their sexual orientation, out-of-school youth, social and economically disadvantaged youth and youth suffering from substance abuse 4. To be reviewed every 5 years 5. Identifies short-term and long-term indicators to assess its impact

(continued)

Table 4.1 (continued)

Sr. No.	Name	Target population	Aim	Launched by	Recommendations for adolescent and youth wellbeing	Key points
5	*National Adolescent Health Strategy 2014*	Adolescents in the age group 10–19 years	To empower adolescents to make well-informed decisions about their health and provide information and services to address various adolescent needs across different sectors and at different levels of care	Ministry of Health and Family Welfare, Govt. of India, and the United Nations Population Fund (UNFPA)	1. Implementing the Rashtriya Kishor Swasthya Karyakram (RKSK) and its components (Sect. 4.3.3) 2. Shifts lens from clinical and treatment focused approach to a wellness approach with focus on health promotion	Has six priority areas: Sexual and reproductive health Violence-free living *Mental and emotional wellbeing* *Prevention of substance misuse* Healthy and disease-free lifestyle Improved nutritional status

Therefore, there is need for specific strategic directions and recommendations to address adolescent and youth mental health nationally. The Mental Health Policy and Service Guidance Package by the World Health Organization, 2005, identifies the need for a policy specific to the context of children and adolescents as a reference for all strategic and programmatic initiatives and implementations targeted towards this group. The need for such a policy specific to a particular group of individuals has been recognised, to ensure a developmental perspective, and to reduce the effects of systemic changes, such as budget cuts on the services for this population (Sharan and Sagar 2007). The National Mental Health Policy also identifies the need for specific policies, laws, regulations, implementation plans and monitoring processes in different sectors (*5.1.1*) to address specific needs and ensure effective implementation of programmes and services. In this view, it is important to deliberate the possibilities of creating a new framework or policy to address mental health needs specific to adolescents and youth. During the consultative meet, one of the experts aptly said, 'Policy making is the art of the possible rather than the art of the necessary'. Policy documents may not always meet the requirements of all groups, and therefore serve primarily as a broad framework that drives programmes and services, thus making it important for the state governments and local bodies to identify specific needs of different groups and address them at a programmatic level while referring to the policy as a guideline. This also makes it necessary for policies to be reviewed in order to evolve with time.

While the process of developing a new policy requires a huge investment of resources, it will require a thorough mapping of adolescent and youth needs and services across different contexts, and that might help tremendously in assessing the current status of adolescent and youth mental health in the country and identifying the needs of this population. Further, it may help in prioritising urgent issues and also facilitate the development of strategies and programmes to address those needs. However, it is important to point out that drafting a new policy will also have to take into account the heterogeneous nature of this group and identify the different needs across different sociocultural contexts within the country. Since most programmes and services addressing mental health needs of adolescents and youth are implemented and delivered at the state level, it is important to question the practical feasibility of investing so many resources in procuring data and creating a national-level framework.

Another possibility is creating a specific set of guidelines for adolescent and youth mental health within the existing policy frameworks, at the national level or at the level of the states. This will ensure representation of specific mental health needs of adolescents and youth within a sociocultural context. An example of a similar adaptation is the Karnataka Youth Policy. This state youth policy aims to address the developmental needs of young people between the ages 16 and 30 years and empower them. Among the many focus areas, the policy also recognises the importance of mental and emotional health of young people and recommends strategies like creating mental health centres and a 24×7 helpline to address mental health concerns of youth. While such a framework may provide directions for mental health services and plans, it will be important to recognise the role of all stakeholders and collaborate with service providers at different levels to ensure effective implementation.

The proposal of including specific guidelines for adolescent and youth mental health within the existing national mental health policy seems more feasible as it will ensure uniformity in the values, philosophy and principles that serve as a benchmark for all strategies and activities. It may also promote inclusion of adolescent- and youth-related initiatives within the broader domain of mental health initiatives and action plans.

4.3 Adolescent and Youth Mental Health-Related Programmes

The policies mentioned above can be translated into action through various programmes addressing adolescent and youth mental health at different levels of care. In the absence of any comprehensive documentation of services for adolescent mental health, this chapter attempts to review programmes across different levels that address adolescent mental health needs. This section will begin with a discussion of the National Mental Health Programme and the District Mental Health Programme, both of which operate under and are monitored by the Ministry of Health and Family Welfare (MoHFW), Government of India, and the Rashtriya Kishor Swasthya Karyakram (RKSK). This will be followed by a review a few programmes and projects across India working in the mental health sector and/or focus on adolescent and youth mental health.

4.3.1 National Mental Health Programme

The National Mental Health Programme (NMHP) was the first national-level programmatic initiative taken by the Government of India in 1982 to address the mental health needs of the population in the country with an aim to create easily available and accessible mental health services for all and the utilisation of mental health knowledge in healthcare services with a focus on community participation and self-help. There is no specific mandate, objective or action plan for adolescents and youth under the NMHP. One of the experts consulted expressed how the NMHP does not identify substance use and suicide as significant psychological disorders in the context of adolescents and youth. The NMHP was revised and re-strategised in 2003 in the 10th five-year plan to provide grants for modernisation of state-run hospitals, upgradation of psychiatric wings in hospitals, establishing centres of excellence and strengthening postgraduate departments of educational institutes. This will be discussed further in Sect. 4.3.2.

4.3.2 *District Mental Health Programme*

The District Mental Health Programme (DMHP) was initiated in 1996 under the NMHP with the objective to integrate mental health with general healthcare and providing community mental health services. The DMHP recognised the significance of adolescent and youth mental health and wellbeing and in its revision during 2011 recognised the need to take a life course perspective to mental health. The DMHP also emphasises the need to implement Life Skills Training programmes by the DMHP team in collaboration with educational institutes or NGOs. The Central Implementation Team has been assigned the task to assess the NIMHANS Life Skills Training module for use across the country and suggest recommendations. In addition, the DMHP identifies the role of teachers as trainers for class 8, 9 and 10 students and identifies school mental health programmes as a potential area of development. According to the Annual Report of the MoHFW for the year 2015–2016, the DMHP is currently extended to 241 districts.

As part of the NMHP re-strategisation by the end of the 10th five-year plan, DMHP was extended to 110 districts, and upgradation of psychiatric wings of 71 medical colleges/general hospitals and modernisation of 23 mental hospitals were funded (Sinha and Kaur 2011). A review of these plans revealed that the programme and aforementioned developments could not be implemented as effectively due to lack of skilled manpower, namely, psychiatrists, social workers and psychologists, lack of monitoring, lack of detailed operational guidelines and lack of coordination between the departments of medical education and health at the state level, among other concerns (Sinha and Kaur 2011).

In 2008, the Indian Council for Market Research (ICMR) reviewed the DMHP in 20 districts, and in 2011 NIMHANS reviewed the DMHP in 23 districts from the four southern states of India. The Policy Group appointed by the MoHFW in 2011 to redesign the DMHP evaluated the DMHP by considering the aforementioned reviews and found that lack of funds, coordination between ministries and departments and differences in the interpretation of objectives and goals across different districts were resulting in the poor functioning of the DMHP. The Policy Group has recommended including child mental health services at district hospitals which will include identification of mental health problems in schoolgoing children through a trained district mental health team and ensure provisions for catering to severe psychological disorders in children through an outpatient service. The Policy Group also recommends including the number of child service users as an outcome indicator for DMHP.

The review of the DMHP in 20 districts (Indian Council for Market Research 2008) identified the need for adequate training of all healthcare professionals working in the DMHP. The Policy Group shares that the training conducted focused on hard skills with little focus on soft skills, personal development or leadership training. At the same time, the role of psychosocial interventions is highly underrepresented in the trainings. The review also highlighted some successful innovations and practices carried out to address needs of schoolgoing children (Policy Group 2012). In the Madurai district, 300 corporation school teachers have been trained in Life Skills Training with a focus on positive mental health, parenting skills and coping with stress, through the help of SHGs. Dr. Mahalakshmi, a psychiatrist in Dindigul district of Tamil Nadu, has initiated an adolescent school mental health programme and imparted training on disabilities in over 300 higher secondary schools (Policy Group DMHP 2012). As part of the school mental health programme, 210 children identfied as requiring psychological support received counselling services in school (Policy Group DMHP 2012). While evidence of the programme's impact is not available, these practices received a mention under 'programmes that work well' by the Policy Group of the DMHP.

4.3.3 Rashtriya Kishor Swasthya Karyakram

The Rashtriya Kishor Swasthya Karyakram (RKSK) was launched by the MoHFW in 2014 to address the needs of adolescents and youth in India. It aims to assist adolescents and youth in maximising their potential by responding to their health and development requirements through seven strategic components (7Cs), namely, coverage, content, communities, clinics, counselling, communication and convergence. While the RKSK focuses on different aspects of adolescent health, two of the most relevant objectives of the RKSK in the context of this chapter are enhancing mental health and preventing substance misuse. The RKSK strategy handbook cites data from epidemiological studies and introduces the spheres of influence on adolescent health (Blum 2005 as cited in RKSK strategy handbook, Government of India, 2014) which identifies depression, suicidal tendencies, mental retardation, eating disorders and substance use as risk factors during adolescence. It mentions the increase of psychological disorders like depression and anxiety during adolescence and the gender disparity that takes place during this period. In order to address these mental health needs of adolescents, the RKSK has identified various strategies including community-based interventions like Peer Education (PE) and Quarterly Adolescent Health Day (AHD) and facility-based interventions such as Adolescent Friendly Health Clinics (AFHCs).

The RKSK lists down specific outcome indicators to assess the impact of the strategies and ground level activities. One of the striking features of the RKSK strategy is the focus on ongoing assessments and surveys to measure the outcomes for each of these objectives. Further, the role of auxiliary nurse midwife (ANM) and teachers in identifying signs of psychological disorders and role of caregivers and peers in reporting substance use have been identified as significant output indicators. The programme has also highlighted the need for convergence with other national- and state-level departments within and beyond the MoHFW. It aims to collaborate with existing programmes such as integrating mental health information with Life Skills Training in the Adolescent Education Programmes (AEP) in schools, screening through Rashtriya Bal Swasthya Karyakram (RBSK), creating awareness in community-based institutions and incorporating adolescent psychological disorders in curriculum of educational institutes. It also aims at collaborating with Sabla (Rajiv Gandhi Scheme for Empowerment of Adolescent Girls) and teen clubs of the Nehru Yuva Kendra Sangathan (NYKS) to address psychological disorders in out-of-school adolescents.

The strategies and interventions under the Adolescent Health Division as part of the RKSK fall broadly into three categories: community-based interventions (PE and AHD), facility-based interventions (AFHCs and counsellors) and communication through the Adolescent Helpline. The nature of services provided to address mental health needs and objectives at the community level and within existing healthcare facilities is represented in Figs. 4.1, 4.2 and 4.3.

RKSK: Current Status

The RKSK strategies seem to be a significant step in addressing the mental health needs of adolescents and youth in India. The Population Council conducted a study to assess the status of AFHCs and the quality of services provided, as perceived by service users as well as service providers like counsellors, ANMs, Accredited Social Health Activists (ASHA) and Medical Officers (MO) in Maharashtra, Jharkhand and Rajasthan. The study found that service users had a positive experience with the healthcare providers who they reported as being attentive and respectful and who did not make fun of them or shout at them (Santhya et al. 2014). They also reported feeling safe about confidentiality of their information. However, service users mentioned the lack of physical, visual and auditory privacy as well as limited consultation time as significant concerns. They also reported that information provided by the healthcare workers was not comprehensive, limited and sometimes judgemental and moralistic. This study therefore highlights the need for uniform

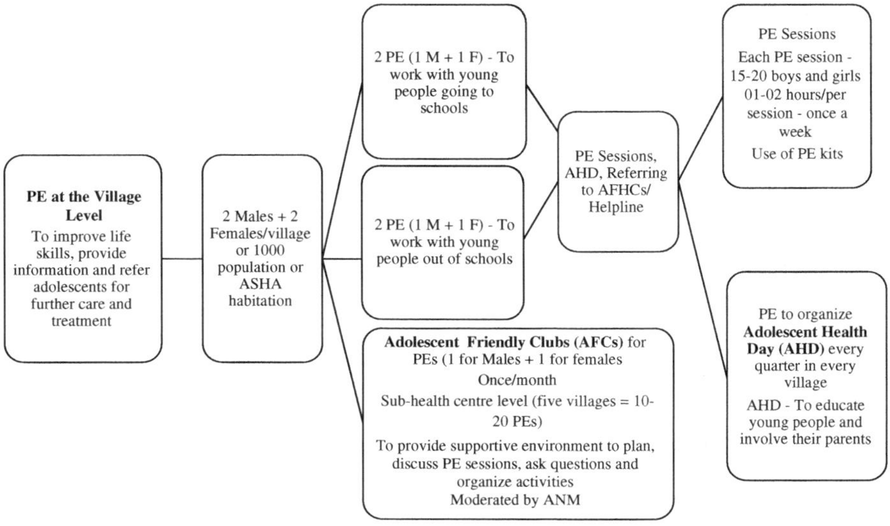

Fig. 4.1 Community-based services provided at the village and sub-centre levels under the RKSK

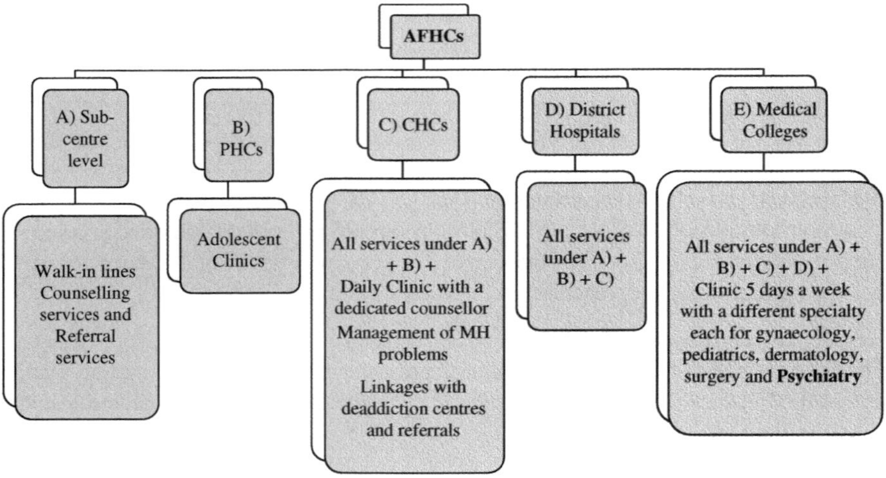

Fig. 4.2 Services provided by the AFHCs at different levels under the RKSK

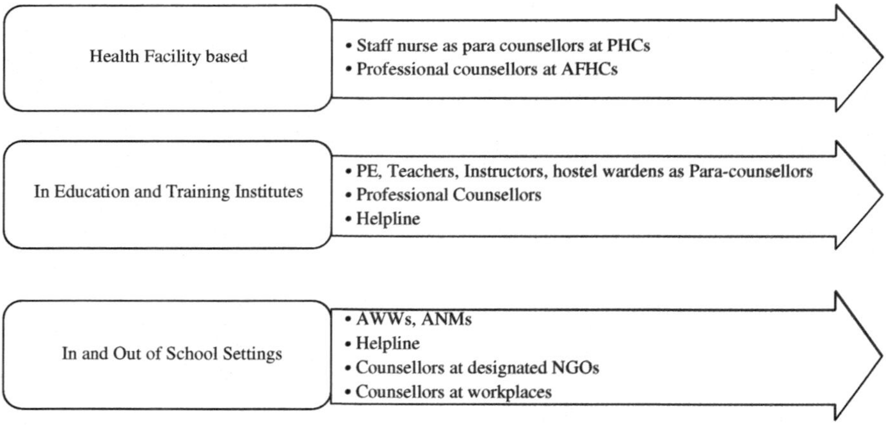

Fig. 4.3 Nature of counselling services at different levels under the RKSK

and quality training for healthcare service providers especially counsellors in the AFHCs on mental health and counselling skills.

According to the Annual Report of the MoHFW 2015–2016, trainings of MOs, ANMs and counsellors have been regular across PHCs and AFHCs. In Maharashtra, the RKSK programme is operational in 9 out of the 36 districts. The state government planned to establish 181 AFHCs during the year 2016–2017. The Maitri clinics provide counselling services and create awareness about mental health through Information Education Communication (IEC) resources. Peer educators are being trained and provided with uniforms and identity cards, and events like Adolescent

Health Days have also been conducted. The need for capacity building of counsellors, empowerment of peer educators, development of more interactive PE session plans and user-friendly IEC material have all been identified as challenges in the effective implementation of the RKSK in Maharashtra.

4.3.4 Other Programmes

In addition to programmes initiated by the Government of India, there are many other adolescent- and youth-oriented mental health programmes operating at different levels in the country. For the purpose of this chapter, a few national, state-level and community-based projects and programmes have been identified, based on recommendations by experts as good practice models. Table 4.2 presents a brief overview of some of these programmes and the activities they conduct to address adolescent and youth mental health needs. This list is not exhaustive and may not be representative of all existing services within this sector.

4.3.5 Research Projects

In addition to programmes on the field, there are many ongoing research projects which aim to study new aspects of adolescent and youth mental health and gain insights in the field.

The research project titled Consortium on Vulnerability to Externalizing Disorders and Addictions [c-VEDA] is a funded project initiated in 2015 under the ICMR-UK Medical Research Centre (MRC) partnership with principal investigators from King's College London and experts from NIMHANS. Given the significant problem of substance use among adolescents, this research project is likely to provide newer insights in substance use among adolescents and youth.

Another research project titled 'Development of Community Child and Adolescent Mental Health Service Model' (NIMHANS 2015) is funded by the Karnataka State Integrated Child Protection Society (KSICPS), an additional managerial body assisting the Department of Women and Child Development, Government of Karnataka. The principal investigator for the project is a senior expert from NIMHANS, and the project has the potential to provide directions in terms of what could be ways of responding to adolescent mental health needs at the community level.

The recently launched SPIRIT project, implemented by the Indian Law Society (ILS) in collaboration with national and international organisations, is supported by the MoHFW and focuses on suicide prevention and mental health intervention in India. The project is a five-year initiative that is aimed at suicide prevention intervention in a community setting.

Table 4.2 List of programmes at various levels addressing adolescent and youth mental health needs

Sr. No.	Name	Target population	Aim	Launched by	Activities
State-level programme					
1	*Yuva Spandana 2014*	Youth in Karnataka	To promote mental health across 10 districts in Karnataka as part of the Karnataka Youth Policy	NIMHANS, funded by the Department of Youth Empowerment and Sports, Govt. of Karnataka	1. Each district would have five Yuva Parivarthakas, all below the age of 35 years who will interact with students in schools and colleges urging them to enrol for the Yuva Mitra programme 2. Yuva Parivarthakas will train 25 Yuva Mitras who will serve as first-line counsellors providing assistance and empathetic listening to students and individuals between the ages 15 and 30 years 3. Project report as of March 2015 highlights the establishment of Yuva Spandana Kendras in 9 districts and having completed 219 sensitisation programmes The programme was officially launched in Karnataka in October 2016
District-level programme					
2	*Police Didi*	Children in schools and communities in Mumbai	To prevent and reduce the cases of child sexual abuse in the city of Mumbai (Mishra A. P. 2016)	Mumbai Commissioner of Police Dattatray Padsalgikar	1. Police Didi is a female police officer who will take on the role of an advocate and visit schools and communities to provide sessions on good and bad touch and keep a check on any suspicious activity around these schools 2. A number of cases being registered under the Protection of Children from Sexual Offences (POCSO) Act have reduced since the initiation of this project as reported

School-based programmes					
3	*PRemIum for aDolEscEnts (PRIDE) 2015*	Adolescents in Goa and Delhi	To identify the treatment gap and address two barriers in effective implementation of psychological treatments for adolescents: lack of trained and skilled human resources and lack of indigenous models and poor 'generalisability' of Western models	Sangath	1. Attempts to develop a psychosocial intervention delivered according to a transdiagnostic stepped-care model to address common mental health needs of adolescents 2. Aims to digitise all the processes and creating e-learning courses
4	*Apni Shala*	State government schools across Mumbai	To promote social emotional learning amongst school children	Apni Shala	1. Develops content and curriculum to help students share personal experiences through creative form of expression like stories, drama, community projects and art 2. Conduct trainings for teachers and counsellors to enable and empower them to facilitate student sessions
Programmes in conflict-affected areas					
5	*Paigaam*	Young individuals in Kashmir	To train, educate and empower youth and children in peacebuilding and peacekeeping skills based on the principles of peace psychology		1. Incorporate peace education within school curriculum and provide training in conflict conciliation, nonviolent communication and mediation and facilitation 2. Provide skills for psychological intervention including mental health counselling, trauma healing, stress management and post-conflict psychological recovery as well as youth leadership development which include career guidance, skills and personality development

(continued)

Table 4.2 (continued)

Sr. No.	Name	Target population	Aim	Launched by	Activities
6	*HELP Foundation 1997*	Young individuals in Jammu and Kashmir	To provide education, empowerment and mental health services like counselling to individuals, especially children affected by the violence and conflict in the valley		1. Set up a mental health institute to provide services for mental healthcare, suicide prevention, drug de-addiction and domestic violence 2. Started a school by the name step by step for children with learning disabilities 3. As part of outreach programmes, doctors conducted mental health awareness programmes with a focus on alcohol and drug addiction in schools and colleges
Working with vulnerable groups					
7	*Koshish 2011*	Homeless people across all age groups	To address issues of homelessness and destitution	TISS	1. Youth Engagement Programme that involves interaction with youth from colleges and universities and helps them recognise the reality of homelessness and enabling them to develop a sense of justice and fairness
8	*Prayas 1990*	Vulnerable groups in Mumbai and Bharuch	To rehabilitate and empower vulnerable groups	Centre for Criminology and Justice, TISS	1. Works with a range of vulnerable groups including youth under trial prisoners and those being processed by the criminal justice system as well as those referred by personnel within the system 2. Team of social workers, vocational instructors and counsellors working at the Youth Development Centre

9	*Project Chunauti 2010*		To strengthen systems for care for children in institutions and rehabilitation and create a model for the same	Centre for Law and Society, TISS	
Web-based and telephonic services					
10	*Virtual Knowledge Network 2014*	Mental health professionals	To provide e-learning modules covering various topics related to addiction and mental health	Centre for Addiction Medicine (CAM), NIMHANS	1. Case discussions and video conferences on substance-induced psychotic disorders, adolescent and addiction, behavioural addiction, substance use in special populations
11	*Karnataka Youth Portal*	Youth in Karnataka	To 'reach, engage and empower' the youth	Govt. of Karnataka	1. Provides information about youth-related activities and aims to engage the youth in social and political activities
12	*White Swan Foundation 2014*	Youth	To provide information on various common and severe mental health disorders, mental health issues as well as rights and legal information	NIMHANS	1. Portal provides detailed understanding of suicide and actions and interventions to be taken to prevent suicide as well as substance use and interventions for the same 2. The style of writing is adolescent friendly and uses different styles of content delivery like videos, articles and comic strips
13	*Initiating Concern for All (iCall) 2011*	Individuals across all age groups	To provide counselling services through telephone and email	TISS, Mumbai	1. The three major areas of focus: telephonic and email counselling, training and outreach activities 2. Adolescents and youth constitute about 10–15% of the total calls received per month and about 20–25% of the total emails received per month

(continued)

Table 4.2 (continued)

Sr. No.	Name	Target population	Aim	Launched by	Activities
Adolescent- and youth-led programmes					
14	*The YP Foundation*	Young people across India	To enable young people to create programmes and influence policies in the areas of sexuality, gender, health, education, governance and arts		1. Life skills, education and health programme for children and adolescents titled 'Blending Spectrum' which aims to engage and train young people as peer educators to provide children and adolescents from lower socio-economic backgrounds with leadership opportunities and increasing their awareness on health and hygiene 2. 2009–2013 – conducted 108 life skills workshops with 40 out-of-school children
15	*Youth Ki Awaaz 2008*	Young people across India	To provide Indian youth with a space to voice their ideas, concerns and thoughts	Indian youth	1. Stories and personal narratives related to mental health ranging from reviews of mental health services offered across the country, critical analysis of laws like the Mental Healthcare Bill, user-survivor narratives, views on suicide, mental health of students and many other adolescent and youth mental health-related topics
16	*Reach Out 2015*	School students	To create awareness about mental health among students and provide a peer-based network to support students	School students in Mumbai	1. Visual campaigns, self-help books, social media, class presentations and monthly campaigns to address specific adolescent mental health issues

4.3.6 *Review of Programmes*

As seen in Table 4.2, there are many programmes implemented at different levels to address the mental health needs of adolescents and young people in India. To present a broad overview on mental health programmes for adolescents and youth, the programmes have been reviewed along the following parameters adapted from the mental health context model provided in the World Health Organization Mental Health Policy and Service Guidance Package (2005): target population, levels of care (promotion, prevention, treatment, rehabilitation), human resources, intersectoral collaboration and monitoring and research.

Most programmes are quite new, and extensive data on the implementation and impact of these programmes is not available in the public domain. However, some programmes have effectively documented their impact and outreach in annual publications. The focus here is not to review each programme and assess impact and outcomes achieved but instead present the reader with the breadth and scope of existing programmes along certain axes.

Target Population
Most of the programmes reviewed are addressing mental health needs of adolescents and youth distinctly. Some programmes focus on populations across all age groups including adolescents and youth. Among the programmes reviewed, while some are specifically designed to address needs of distinct groups such as vulnerable adolescents, schoolgoing adolescents and students at risk for sexual abuse, etc., there are some with a focus on providing interventions for all mental health needs of adolescents. While the national-level programmes seem to provide a comprehensive package for all adolescent needs, many groups requiring special focus are not highlighted within the same. For instance, needs of adolescents experiencing sexual abuse are not prominently identified in these programmes. This indicates the need to redesign the national-level programmes to identify needs of specific groups within the larger population of adolescents. Additionally, while many programmes are addressing schoolgoing children, not many services are available for out-of-school adolescents or adolescents in institutions. This is also an important area requiring attention from the service delivery sector.

Levels of Care: Promotion, Prevention, Treatment, and Rehabilitation
An important factor in reviewing mental health programmes is the level of care at which the programme aims to provide services. From the programmes reviewed, it is essential to observe that some programmes are working to promote mental health and prevent mental illness among adolescents and youth. One such example is the Life Skills Education (LSE) programme conducted through national- and state-level programmes and community-based organisations. These LSE programmes help reach out to large numbers of adolescents and youth within and beyond schools and colleges. In addition to the organizations enlisted in Table 4.2, many organizations like Pratham, Kaivalya Education Foundation, Dream a Dream and Magic Bus have been providing life skills development programmes for adolescents from vulnerable

and underpriviledged backgrounds Some programmes are designed to provide interventions to those experiencing mental distress. It is also important to note that there is an absence of nationwide programmes for mental health advocacy and promotion. This highlights the need for advocacy-based initiatives for adolescents and young people in the country.

Human Resources
This is an important factor in understanding the roles played by different professionals and the capacities built through various programmes. As observed in Table 4.2, programmes like *Yuva Spandana* (Spandana 2015) and other youth-led programmes are strengthening capacities of adolescents and youth and developing the potential of the youth in India. Other programmes like *Police Didi* and *Apnishala* (Apnishala, n.d.) are utilising existing human resources and training them to address mental health needs of young people. Training community workers and first-line respondents helps reduce the mental health service burden on specialists and ensures that services are provided effectively and immediately to those in need. The third group of organisations which provide mental health interventions mainly through telephonic- and web-based services often involve mental health professionals for service delivery. However, the training received by these professionals in addressing adolescent-specific concerns is not documented. This is an important area of future research to identify the skills required by professionals working with adolescents and designing training curriculum for the same.

Intersectoral Collaboration
One aspect about mental health programmes that has been discussed under the National Mental Health Policy as well as the RKSK, and also recommended by various experts, is a focus on collaboration and convergence. Most effective practices require strong associations with partnering organisations from public and private sector for implementation of the action plans. Similarly, private and non-profit organisations also require to partner and provide support to existing government programmes to strengthen mental healthcare systems at the community and district level and to ensure quality service provision across all levels. Since adolescents and young people are embedded within various sociocultural contexts, it is important for programmes to identify the impact of these micro and macro systems on adolescent wellbeing. One such example is the utilisation of schools and colleges as platforms for adolescent mental health advocacy and prevention.

Monitoring and Research
It is important for programmes delivering services to carry out research and provide findings from the field. Such data is useful in understanding the mental health needs of adolescents and young people and the services required. Similarly, monitoring the programmes and conducting regular assessments is essential to understand the impact and outreach of the programmes. For instance, the project report for *Yuva*

Spandana provides a glimpse into the effectiveness of the programme and the probable scope of the programme in the near future.

Therefore, while adolescent- and youth-related mental health programmes are effectively operating across the country, it is important to bring together these dedicated efforts, consolidate the initiatives and further expand and scale them to create an effective integrated system of services and programmes that can reach maximum individuals.

4.4 Convergence of Adolescent and Youth Mental Health-Related Policies and Programmes

The need for coordination between mental health services provided by departments and ministries has been acknowledged by the Mental Health Care Act 2017. Under clause 32 in chapter VI 'Duties of the Government' of the Act, the responsibility of the Government to ensure coordination between all services provided under the areas of health, law, home affairs, human justice, social justice, employment, education, women and child development, and medical education has been emphasised in order to address mental health needs of the population. This is further evident in the representation of different ministries and departments in the composition of the Central Mental Health Authority as established by the Central Government under clause 33 of the Act to ensure development of mental health services, training, supervisions and delivery of services. The RKSK also highlights the significance of working with other departments and ministries in addressing needs of adolescents and youth by assessing the status of other relevant departments and programmes, identifying possible areas of convergence, assessing possible obstacles and amenability of other programmes and gaining approval from the District/State Committee for Adolescent Health (DCAH/SCAH) for the same. The RKSK operational handbook mentions different programmes under various ministries which can assist in achieving its objectives and in the delivery of services. It mentions the role of the NMHP under the MoHFW and its linkages with the DMHP and psychiatric wings of medical colleges for referral purposes.The RKSK also recognises the role of National Rural Health Mission (NRHM) in addition to other programmes and agencies in guiding the provess of outcome assessment of the programme. The National Youth Policy also identifies that services and programmes addressing mental health needs of adolescents and youth are fragmented and recommends developing a framework to ensure coordinated efforts by identifying the existing stakeholders, evaluating the quality of services and providing a platform to align these efforts. The need for collaboration has also been highlighted in the National Mental Health Policy 2014 under intersectoral collaboration, which emphasises the need for partnerships between government (public) and non-government (private and non-profit) sectors.

The RKSK and DMHP also align with sub-clause (a) of sub-section (5) of clause 18 of the Mental Health Care Act which calls for integration of mental health services with general healthcare services at primary, secondary and tertiary levels. This is also outlined in one of the principles of the National Mental Health Policy 2014, which mentions that mental health services are to be provided within the existing healthcare system by adopting the primary healthcare approach. The RKSK recognizes the role of integrating training required for adolescent health programmes with existing training for other departments of the MoHFW instead of parallel training sessions, as well as including it as part of undergraduate and postgraduate medical and nursing courses. The National Adolescent Health Strategy which forms the framework for the RKSK is found to converge with the philosophy and the five strategic prongs of the UNFPA's Global Adolescent and Youth Strategy 2012–2013 (UNFPA 2013). The common elements include focus on sexuality and reproductive health services, evidence-based practices, adolescent and youth leadership (seen through PE programmes under RKSK), Life Skills Education and community trainers. The National Youth Policy also identifies these as significant domains for youth development. The Policy, under its objective to create a strong and healthy future generation, identifies the need to address emotional and mental health issues such as depression and risk for suicide. The Policy also mentions the need to create a targeted awareness and outreach programme to address the youth at risk, which is in line with the initiatives carried out by the RKSK through AHD and PE sessions.

The RKSK provides a comprehensive framework to address the need for convergence. It proposes the formation of a Steering Committee for Adolescent Health and Development (SCAHD) at the national level, the State Committee for Adolescent Health (SCAH) at the state level and the District Committee for Adolescent Health (DCAH) at the district level, all of which will implement convergence-related strategies in collaboration with the existing Village Health, Nutrition and Sanitation Committees (VHNSCs) at the village level. The DMHP districts in Kerala and Tamil Nadu are exceptions demonstrating the positive influence of intra- and intersectoral coordination at the state level. In Maharashtra, one of the experts reported that there is a large scope for convergence between the existing programmes at ground level such as referral of schoolgoing children and adolescents from the RKSK to the DMHP for specialised care and services. While such systems are in practice in a few districts, he informed that there is lack of consistent efforts in this direction. A detailed review of the functioning of these various committees across different states will provide insights into the status on convergence and the challenges faced in the process.

The DMHP, RKSK, Mental Health Care Act 2017 and the National Mental Health Policy 2014 are also aligned in their ethos as evident in their overlapping value systems. The DMHP aims to take a life course perspective, adopting an equity lens, ensuring evidence-based practices in a rights-based manner through a health systems perspective. The Mental Health Care Act 2017 has also listed quality-based care, promotion of principles of active participation, efficiency and equity as well as protecting rights and dignity of the individual as its basic objectives. The National Mental Health Policy too adopts an equity lens while providing quality, evidence-based, holistic care through a participatory, integrated and rights-based approach. The key principles of the RKSK, similar to the National Adolescent Health Strategy which guides the programme, are gender equity, inclusion, participation, rights and strategic partnerships. These intersections in the philosophical guidelines provide for a basic framework to establish the strategies for convergence.

Mental healthcare services are a vast sector of healthcare encompassing medical, social, political and rehabilitative needs of the individual. These needs are distinct from one another and addressed by different administrative bodies at different levels of healthcare. While this process of shared responsibility allows for specialised care, its success is contingent on a well-synchronised system of different ministries and departments. As mentioned above, the need for intra- and intersectoral collaboration has been identified at the policy and programmatic levels. While some initiatives in this direction have already been taken at different levels, most activities and programmes at the national and state level seem to be implemented independently.

The review conducted by the Policy Group appointed by the MoHFW in 2011 highlights the lack of coordination between Ministries in responding to the mental health needs of the population. This has a negative impact on the delivery of comprehensive and quality mental health services to those in need. In a striking example, the Policy Group identifies the lack of intersectoral coordination between the rehabilitation services to be provided by the Ministry of Social Justice and Empowerment and mental health services which come under the purview of the MoHFW. The review also identifies a similar pattern at the state and district levels. For instance, the implementation of DMHP has been negatively impacted by the lack of coordination between the Directorate of Medical Education which looks into the Psychiatry Departments in Government Medical Colleges and the Directorate of Public Health which looks after the PHCs. At the district levels, the lack of incentives for teaching professionals to work at PHCs and the exclusion of mental health from the NRHM's agenda have also been cited as severe limitations. In the area of child mental healthcare, the missing links are observed in the division of services between different ministries. For instance, the review mentions that services for children with disabilities are managed by the Ministry of Social Justice and Empowerment and school counselling services are provided by Ministry of Human Resource Development.

The review report also highlights the need for a central and state-level monitoring system and periodic reviews to ensure accountability of the services provided. Interestingly, the Health Management Information System set up by the NRHM has not included mental health, thereby not accounting for mental healthcare services provided to the community. This makes it difficult to map the existing services in the mental health sector and to assess and evaluate the same. These observations demand for more communication and better coordination among various departments and sectors of service provision.

4.5 Recommendations

The above review of policies and programmes offers an overview of the strengths and challenges of the existing provisions for adolescents and youth in India to address their mental health needs. In light of this review, this chapter also attempts to provide a brief list of recommendations across four priority areas of action – research, policy, programmes and advocacy. Strategic recommendations under each of these will be discussed in this section. Table 4.3 presents these strategies in the context of the priority areas of action to effectively strengthen the policies and programmatic services for adolescent and youth wellbeing.

Table 4.3 Areas of action and strategic recommendations

Sr. No.	Area of action	Strategies
1.	*Research*	Review existing national/international policies and programmes to identify guidelines and best practices
		Conduct outcome research to identify the efficacy and effectiveness of mental health services across all national-level programmes
2.	*Policy*	Draft policy briefs and share them with adolescents, youth and other stakeholders
		Develop adolescent and youth mental health-related guidelines
3.	*Programmes*	Provide skill-based training to counsellors, healthcare professionals and community workers for screening and early identification of psychological disorders, counselling adolescents, specialised interventions for different psychological disorders
		Develop pilot projects such as an urban AFHC and School Mental Health Programme to address mental health needs of adolescents and youth in the community
		Monitor and review existing mental health programmes for adolescents and youth
		Develop mental health outcome indicators for programme evaluation in the Indian context
		Conduct regular consultations with various stakeholders to further convergence and collaboration
4.	*Advocacy*	Create spaces for and encourage adolescent- and youth-led initiatives
		Use technology effectively to create awareness on mental health and promote wellbeing of adolescents and youth

4.5.1 Research

The existing reviews of policies in India often exist in the form of annual reports or reviews conducted at regular intervals by the ministry overseeing the policy. Programmes, on the other hand, are reviewed based on existing outcome indicators to assess the larger impact. However, this data and reports are not reviewed alongside international standards and very rarely are user voices highlighted in these reviews. It is important therefore to conduct comprehensive reviews of policies and programmes using appropriate methodology and in light of existing literature and epidemiological data. It is also important to acknowledge that many of these policies need to be reviewed and revised after regular intervals in light of changing social and cultural trends so that the relevance of the policies and the effectiveness of the programmes are achieved.

Conduct Outcome Research to Identify the Efficacy and Effectiveness of Mental Health Services Across All National-Level Programmes
While there are many national-level programmes like the RKSK offering counselling services to individuals and programmes like the DMHP which offer mental healthcare, it is important to assess these services and identify their strengths. Timely reviews, administering outcome rating scales, feedback from service users, exit interviews and consultations with service providers will help identify the effectiveness of various services and improve the same.

Review Existing National/International Policies and Programmes to Identify Guidelines and Best Practices
This chapter has briefly reviewed the Indian policies relevant to adolescent and youth mental health. Future research can aim to review other relevant policies and acts including the Protection of Children from Sexual Offences (POCSO), the Juvenile Justice Act (2005), the policy on substance use, alcohol prevention policy, UGC regulations in curbing the menace of ragging in higher educational institutes (2009) and laws for cybercrime including cyber bullying, among others. One of the experts suggested conducting a meta-analysis of all these policies and identifying their commonalities, distinctions and limitations. Similarly, reviews of international policies and legal documents will help in strengthening the existing systems in India. Selected elements from the international guidelines can be adapted to suit the Indian context. Best practice models and services from around the world can also be reviewed critically to identify strategies that can enhance the efficacy of programmes in India.

4.5.2 Policy

As pointed out in Sect. 4.2.3, there is an impending need to create policy-level amendments to identify and include adolescents and youth as specific target groups with unique needs and service requirements. One of the experts proposed the idea of creating 'guiding action plans' to supplement the existing policies and implementing the same. It is important therefore to advocate for a special clause on adolescent and youth mental health within existing policy frameworks.

Draft Policy Briefs and Share Them with Adolescents, Youth and Other Stakeholders
User-friendly policy briefs, preferably in local languages, highlighting the components relevant to adolescent and youth mental health can be circulated during outreach activities as part of national- and state-level and community-based programmes and can be uploaded online on youth portals and social media pages. These policy briefs can also be shared with schools and stakeholders like teachers and school management teams and other key stakeholders who can play a critical role in the prevention and promotion of adolescent and youth mental health. Adolescents and youth who are aware of these existing policies can contribute by offering recommendations to strengthen the same.

Develop Adolescent and Youth Mental Health-Related Guidelines
While the need for a new policy for adolescent and youth mental health continues to be debated, policy-makers and community leaders can collaborate to create guidelines to develop effective mental healthcare for adolescents and youth with psychological disorders. This can also be done by consulting professionals from the mental health sector, representatives from the government and young individuals and mental health advocates who can review existing programmes and services and their impact assessment data and develop protocols to address the gap between policy mandates and programmatic actions.

4.5.3 Programmes

As discussed in Sect. 4.3, there are a wide range of well-designed programmes in India at different levels. However, as identified in Sects. 4.3 and 4.4, concerns like lack of skilled manpower, poor coordination and convergence between departments and ministries and lack of supervision prevent effective implementation of these programmes. The need to establish a nodal agency that can assist national- and state-level programmes, initiate and strengthen partnerships with state governments and positively impact programme implementation has been expressed during the consultative meets.

Provide Skill-Based Training to Counsellors, Healthcare Professionals and Community Workers for Screening and Early Identification of Psychological Disorders, Counselling Adolescents and Specialised Interventions for Different Psychological Disorders

The dearth of mental healthcare professionals in India makes it imperative to train community workers and healthcare professionals in counselling and other mental healthcare processes. For counsellors working in the AFHCs and DMHP, it is essential to receive skill-based training in early identification of mental health concerns and specialised interventions and counselling skills for adolescent- and youth-specific psychological disorders.

Develop Pilot Projects such as an Urban AFHC and School Mental Health Programme to Address Mental Health Needs of Adolescents and Youth in the Community

During the consultative meet, experts from the RKSK team mentioned that the AFHCs had received more prominence in rural areas. Developing a model urban AFHC will not only help address these gap but also provide a better understanding of adolescent and youth concerns and help-seeking behaviours in urban areas. Execution of such a project will involve mobilisation of various resources along with context-specific designing of IEC resources and training of healthcare professionals to suit the urban scenario.

The number of schoolgoing adolescents is very high in India and so are the rates of reported psychological disorders among schoolgoing adolescents. It is important therefore to address the psychological wellbeing of these young people in schools. The need for school-based mental health programmes has been expressed in the RKSK, National Mental Health Policy and by the Policy Group of the DMHP (2012). The LSE programmes that are being conducted in communities and schools across many villages and state government schools are not uniformly designed, and the impact of these has not been regularly assessed. One of the experts from NIMHANS recommends establishing specific outcome indicators for LSE programmes and broadening its scope to include lifestyle-enhancing elements like yoga within its purview. Initiating a school mental health programme which promotes adolescent and youth mental health can be implemented across various schools as a pilot project to assess the response from schools and the impact on student wellbeing.

Monitor and Review Existing Programmes

While the ministries review different programmes at regular intervals, it is important for external agencies to monitor and review these programmes too. In addition to national-level programmes like RKSK and DMHP, the impact of various other programmes and services can also be assessed to identify best practices and models across the country.

Develop Mental Health Outcome Indicators for Programme Evaluation in the Indian Context

The impact indicators of most national-level programmes are not robust and do not measure culturally relevant aspects of mental healthcare services. It is essential therefore to develop practical, measurable mental health outcome indicators that are contextually relevant. For instance, measuring the rate of perceived stigma associated with mental health and discrimintion among adolescents, number of trained mental health professionals implementing the programme, rate of suicides or suicidal attempts reported within a district or healthcare centre, number of adolescents identified as requiring mental health suppot, number of adolescents currently receiving mental health treatment, rates of readmission and relapse for adolescents and youth who use substances, measuring changes in rates of school drop-outs and unemployment due to mental illness, etc. can be some of the indicators to assess the quality and impact of various ongoing mental health programmes in the country. In addition to this, mental health outcome indicators across international programmes can be reviewed and adopted after suitable modifications.

Conduct Regular Consultations with Various Stakeholders to Initiate Convergence and Collaboration
In order to strengthen the existing systems, it is important to engage experts from various backgrounds and fields to discuss and brainstorm ideas and plans. Universities and other organisations can create common spaces and invite representatives from the government and other stakeholders in regular consultations to assess the efficiency of various programmes and their effectiveness. These discussions can help in generating suggestions for future action plans and can sensitise officials and field practitioners to various adolescent and youth mental health needs. The chapter proposes the need to facilitate collaboration between governmental, non-governmental sectors and other institutions and partners. A senior government official mentioned that the RKSK is currently not reaching out to secondary schools and colleges and emphasised the need to involve teachers and professors and collaborate with the Department of Education to implement the programme effectively. This would require creating plans for convergence establishing communication systems between different stakeholders.

4.5.4 Advocacy

Adolescents and young individuals can be strong advocates for their own mental health. Involving them in advocacy and outreach and making information and data easily accessible to them will encourage them to be actively engaged in promoting and enhancing their mental health.

Create Spaces for and Encourage Adolescent- and Youth-Led Initiatives
Adolescents and youth are often left out of conversations pertaining to their mental health and wellbeing. It is important to involve them and acknowledge their agency and rights too. This can be done by developing spaces for non-judgemental and non-condescending conversations about mental health. Such practices will encourage young individuals to discuss their concerns and empower them to seek help. One of

the experts shared a personal experience of initiating a peer support group for individuals experiencing bipolar disorder and their caregivers and highlighted the role of such spaces in balancing the power between users and service providers. This space was referred to as the 'fifth space' following the spaces of family, friends, school and leisure, which can assist in harnessing inner resilience and shift perspective from problem-solving to facilitation and support.

Use Technology Effectively to Address Mental Health Needs and Enhance Wellbeing of Adolescents and Youth
Some of the programmes reviewed in the Sect. 4.3 of the chapter have effectively used technology for service delivery to adolescents and youth. Organisations and programmes like the DMHP can create audio-visual content that can be used to facilitate outreach sessions in urban schools and colleges. Academicians and researchers can contribute by developing online courses, podcasts and content to educate young people and empower them to make informed decisions and choices. The use of Information Communication Technology (ICT) to address mental health needs of young people was strongly recommended by various experts during the consultative meet. A senior-level representative from the state government emphasised the role of smartphones, media and social media in information dissemination. Easily downloadable IEC material can be made available on various web-based platforms and social media sites as well as youth portals. Developing mental healthcare apps which can be downloaded on mobile phones is also a great ways to reach out to larger numbers. The UNFPA has launched an App called 'Saathiya Salaah' in 2015 through which peer educators provide information about all adolescent- and youth-related issues including healthcare. While technology can target a larger group of individuals, it is important to recognise the gender imbalance in access to technology. During the consultative meet, a senior central government official highlighted this disparity by pointing out that girls, particularly in northern India, often do not have access or have limited access to technology. While technology driven advocacy can be initiated, outreach through other mediums is equally important in our context.

4.6 Conclusion

The policy frameworks in India seem to address adolescent and youth mental health in some significant ways though not with a special focus. The guidelines for adolescent and youth mental healthcare are not specifically outlined and do not find special mention in most legal and policy documents. The programmes on the other hand seem to be geared towards providing mental healthcare services to adolescents and youth across various settings and different levels of care. However, there are no uniform guidelines for these programmes, and their impact has not been effectively assessed. This chapter provides a bird's eye view of various policies and a few selected programmes. In the light of increasing prevalence of psychological disorders among adolescents and youth, it is important to strengthen the policy recommendations and frameworks that could serve as a strong foundation for the implementation of programmes. This can be followed by more discussion and collaborative planning towards an adolescent and youth mental health policy and programme guidelines that would ensure mental healthcare for all.

Acknowledgements We would like to thank all the officials from the Ministry of Health and Family Welfare, Government of India; representatives from the State Government of Maharashtra; representatives from the RKSK programme; policy-makers and experts who participated in the consultative meet; experts from the National Institute of Mental Health and Neurosciences (NIMHANS), Bengaluru; practicing mental health professionals; and faculty at the Tata Institute of Social Sciences Mumbai for their invaluable inputs and recommendations.

References

(n.d.). Retrieved August 2016, from Paigaam: A Message for Peace: http://www.paigaampeace.org/paigaam-shehjaar-bazaar.html

(n.d.). Retrieved from Virtual Knowledge Network - NIMHANS: http://vlc.nimhans.ac.in/

(n.d.). Retrieved September 2016, from The Y P Foundation: http://www.theypfoundation.org/

(n.d.). Retrieved from White Swan Foundation: http://www.whiteswanfoundation.org/

(n.d.). Retrieved from Karnataka Youth Portal, Department of Youth Empowerment and Sports, Govt. of Karnataka: http://www.karnatakayouthportal.in/

(n.d.). Retrieved September 2016, from Youth Ki Awaaz: http://www.youthkiawaaz.com/

Apnishala. (n.d.). Impact. Retrieved 2016, from Apnishala: http://www.apnishala.org/impact.html.

Adolescent Health Division, Ministry of Health and Family Welfare, Government of India. (2014, January). RKSK Operational Framework – Translating strategy into programmes.

Adolescent Health Division, Ministry of Health and Family Welfare, Government of India. (2015). Guidelines for Implementation of RKSK. New Delhi.

Arun, P., & Chavan, B. (2009). Stress and suicidal ideas in adolescent students in Chandigarh. *Indian Journal of Medical Sciences, 63*(7), 281–287.

Chandrashekarappa, S. M., Ramakrishnaiah, N. M., Ram, D., & Manjunath, R. (2016). Mental Health among adolescent girls - an effort to know the association of mental disorders with socio-demographic variables. *International Journal of Medical Science and Public Health, 5*(11).

Consortium on Vulnerability to Externalizing Disorders and Addictions [c-VEDA]. (n.d.). Retrieved October 2016, from Research Councils UK: http://gtr.rcuk.ac.uk/projects?ref=MR/N000390/1

Department of Health and Family Welfare, Ministry of Health and Family Welfare, Government of India. (2016). *Annual Report 2015–16.* MOHFW.

FundaMentalSDG. (2005). *Position Paper: Mental Health Indicators for the UN Sustainable Development Goals (SDGs).* Retrieved September 2016, from http://www.fundamentalsdg.org/

Gaur, A. D., Vohra, A., Subash, S., & Khurana, H. (2003). Prevalence of psychiatric morbidity among 6 to 14 years old children. *Indian Journal of Community Medicine, 28*(3), 133–137.

Goel, D., Subramanyam, A., & Kamath, R. (2013). A study on the prevalence of internet addiction and its association with psychopathology in Indian adolescents. *Indian Journal of Psychiatry, 55*(2), 140–143. https://doi.org/10.4103/0019-5545.111451.

Government of India. (2017). *The mental healthcare act 2017.* Government of India Ministry of Law and Justice. Retrieved from https://www.prsindia.org/uploads/media/Mental%20Health/Mental%20Healthcare%20Act,%202017.pdf.

Indian Council for Market Research. (2008). *Evaluation of district mental health Prograamme - final report submitted to Ministry of Health and Family Welfare*. Indian Council for Market Research. Retrieved from https://mhpolicy.files.wordpress.com/2011/05/evaluation-of-dmhp-icmr-report-for-the-ministry-of-hfw.pdf.

Mental Health Services. (n.d.). Retrieved September 2016, from HELP Foundation: http://www.jkhf.in/

Ministry of Health and Family Welfare, Government of India. (2004, January). RKSK Strategy Handbook. New Delhi.

Ministry of Health and Family Welfare, Government of India. (2011–12). *Regional Workshops on National Mental Health Programme – A Report.*

Ministry of Health and Family Welfare, Government of India. (2014, October). New Pathways New Hope: National Mental Health Policy of India.

Ministry of Women and Child Development, Government of India. (2013). *The National Policy for Children 2013.*

Ministry of Youth Affairs and Sports, Government of India. (2014). *National Youth Policy 2014.*

Miranda, J. J., & Patel, V. (2005, October). Achieving the millennium development goals: Does mental health play a role? *PLOS Medicine, 2*(10), 0962–0965.

Mishra, A. P. (2016, August 28). *Mumbai slum women and girls find friends in 'Police didi'.* Retrieved August 2016, from The Indian Express: http://indianexpress.com/article/trending/trending-in-india/mumbai-slums-women-girls-find-friends-in-police-didi-3000779/

National Sample Survey Organisation, Ministry of Statistics and Programme Implementation, Government of India. (2002). *NSS 58th round (July–December 2002).* Government of India.

NIMHANS. (2015). *Community Child & Adolescent Mental Health Service Project 2nd quarterly report, January to March 2015.* Dept. of Child & Adolescent Psychiatry, NIMHANS Supported by Dept. of Women & Child Development, Government of Karnataka. Retrieved from http://www.nimhanschildproject.in/reports/.

Office of the Registrar General and Census Commissioner, Ministry of Home Affairs, Government of India. (2011). *Census of India.* Retrieved August 2016, from Population Enumeration Data (Final Population): http://www.censusindia.gov.in/2011census/population_enumeration.html

Patil, R. N., Nagaonkar, S. N., Shah, N. B., & Bhat, T. S. (2013). A cross-sectional study of common psychiatric morbidity in children aged 5–14 years in an urban slum. *Journal of Family Medicine and Primary Care*, 165–168.

Pillai, A., Patel, V., Cardozo, P., Goodman, R., Weiss, H. A., & Andrew, G. (2008). Non-traditional lifestyles and prevalence of mental disorders in adolescents in Goa, India. *The British Journal of Psychiatry, 192*, 45–51.

Policy Group. (2012). *XIIth Plan District Mental Health Programme*. Retrieved from https://mhpolicy.files.wordpress.com/2012/07/final-dmhp-design-xii-plan2.pdf

Prayas. (n.d.). Retrieved 2016, from Tata Institute of Social Sciences: http://www.tiss.edu/view/11/projects/prayas/

PRIDE Progress Half Yearly Report Number 1. (2016). Retrieved September 2016, from Mental Health Innovation: https://mhinnovation.net/sites/default/files/downloads/innovation/reports/PRIDE%20PROGRESS%20HALF%20YEARLY%20REPORT%20NUMBER%201.pdf

Project Chunauti. (n.d.). Retrieved from Tata Institute of Social Sciences: http://tiss.edu/view/11/projects/all-projects/chunauti/

Reddy, B. K., Biswas, A., & Rao, H. (2011). Assessment of mental health of Indian adolescents studying in urban schools. *Malaysian Journal of Paediatrics and Child Health Online Early*.

Santhya, K. G., Prakash, R., Jejeebhoy, S. J., & Singh, S. (2014). *Accessing adolescent friendly health clinics in India: The perspectives of adolescents and youth.* New Delhi: Population Council.

Sharan, P., & Sagar, R. (2007). Mental health policy for children and adolescents in developing countries. *Journal of Indian Association for Child and Adolescent Mental Health, 3*(1), 1–4.

Sinha, S. K., & Kaur, J. (2011). National mental health programme: Manpower development scheme of eleventh five-year plan. *Indian Journal of Psychiatry, 53*(3), 261–265.

Spandana - Developing and implementing district youth mental health promotion services in 10 districts of Karnataka through a district empowerment model – A Karnataka Youth Policy Initiative. (2015). Retrieved from National Institute of Mental Health and Neurosciences: http://nimhans.ac.in/spandana-developing-and-implementing-district-youth-mental-health-promotion-services-10-districts

The Lancet. (2016). *Our future: A lancet commission on adolescent health and wellbeing*. The Lancet.

Thornicroft, G., & Votruba, N. (2015, May). Millennium development goals: lessons for global mental health. *Epidemiology and Psychiatric Sciences*, 1–3.

UNFPA. (2013). *UNFPA strategy on adolescents and youth*. UNFPA. Retrieved from https://www.unfpa.org/sites/default/files/resource-pdf/UNFPA%20Adolescents%20and%20Youth%20Strategy.pdf.

World Health Organization (WHO). (2005). *Mental health policy and service guidance package: Child and adolescent mental health policies and plans*. Geneva: World Health Organization.

World Health Organization. (2014). *Preventing suicide: A global imperative*. Geneva: World Health Organization.

Chapter 5
What Do We Know About Sexual and Reproductive Health of Adolescents and Youth in India: A Synthesis of Literature

M. Sivakami and Saurabh Rai

Abstract Sexual and reproductive health (SRH) is an important facet of the life of young people. Empowering them with the right knowledge and instilling the right attitude during this phase would guarantee lesser vulnerabilities and better health outcomes in their future. This chapter explores the various thematic areas within SRH and synthesises evidence regarding what is known about young people's SRH issues. The research gaps emanating from the literature are described, and the barriers faced by young people in seeking health services for SRH issues have been delineated within the socioecological model. Conducting research among young people is filled with challenges which have been elucidated with the insights gained from conducting key informant interviews with researchers and experts in SRH of young people. There are multiple policies, programmes and laws in India which focus on the sexual and reproductive health of young people. The provisions made under these policies, programmes and laws are critically examined in this chapter to highlight the gaps in them. Through a comprehensive inquiry in the area of SRH of young people based on the existing literature, a deeper understanding of the issue is developed, and recommendations are made to guide policies, programmes and laws to help improve SRH status of young people.

Keywords Adolescents · Youth · Reproductive health · Sexual health · India · Review

---

M. Sivakami (✉)
Center for Health and Social Sciences, School of Health Systems Studies,
Tata Institute of Social Sciences, Mumbai, India
e-mail: sivakami@tiss.edu

S. Rai
School of Health Systems Studies, Tata Institute of Social Sciences, Mumbai, India

S. Bharat, G. Sethi (eds.), *Health and Wellbeing of India's Young People*,
https://doi.org/10.1007/978-981-13-6593-5_5

5.1 Introduction

Adolescence is an important stage in life as it is a transitional phase from childhood to adulthood. It is a time when many factors such as social, economic, biological and demographic play a role in setting the stage for adult life (Population Council and UNICEF 2013). It is estimated that 19.2% (231 million) of the population in India is aged between 15 and 24 years and 20.9% (253 million) are adolescents, i.e. within the age group of 10–19 years (Office of Registrar General of India 2011). This means that one third of India's population is 'young', translating into larger workforce in the future thus leading to greater economic growth and development of the country in long term. It is imperative that this age group realises its full potential which can be ensured with better health, education and productive and livelihood opportunities for them. With the Sustainable Development Goals (SDGs) introduced in 2015 (UN General Assembly Resolution 2015), India needs to invest a lot more on adolescents and young people in order to achieve the goals and capitalise on the demographic dividend that this age group offers.

Until recently, the focus of major government policies has been on children between 0 and 6 years and the reproductive age group of 15–49 years, especially females in the context of pregnancy and motherhood. However, adolescents and youth as a group has started receiving attention recently considering the potential of demographic dividend. The government has been showing great interest in youth, evident from the emphasis in the National Youth Policy 2014 on addressing issues related to livelihood, skills development, marginalisation of rural and tribal youth, sexual and reproductive health, nutrition and others. The Rashtriya Kishor Swasthya Karyakram (RKSK) 2014 implemented as a nationwide programme to address the issues of 10–19 age group, further testifies this. Despite these efforts, there is a need for still greater political commitment to address the needs of the young population.

India's adolescents now may be healthier and better educated, with age at marriage increasing and right to education becoming a reality, but they still face a multitude of barriers in terms of limited access to resources, education, life skills and employment and sexual and reproductive health services. Inequities exist among young people based on their geographical location, cultural context, religion, socio-economic status and marital status which affect their transitioning from adolescence to adulthood and realising their full potential. Hence, it is essential to do synthesis of available evidence from sexual and reproductive health (SRH) research and programmes and policies related to adolescents and young population in India. The objectives of this paper are to review existing evidence and programmes and policies on SRH of adolescents and youth, identify research and programmatic gaps and highlight challenges in carrying out research for adolescents and youth in particular.

In this chapter, individuals between 10 and 19 years have been identified as adolescents, 15–24 years as youth, and collectively from 10 to 24 years as 'young people' (Secretary-General's Report to the General Assembly 1981). This synthesis of literature is based on published articles and unpublished reports from 2001 to

2018. Articles were sourced through several databases (PubMed, Google Scholar, J-Gate, Web of Science, JSTOR and Scopus) and websites of the UNFPA, WHO, UNICEF and Population Council. The articles were chosen based on clarity in objectives and description of study settings, acknowledging limitations to ensure quality. Abstracts were used if full text was not available. Policies, programmes and laws related to SRH were examined through government documents and reports available on websites of different departments and ministries without a time frame. Programme and policy evaluations and critiques of laws and amendments were actively searched to get different perspectives. Large-scale studies such as the National Family Health Survey (NFHS), District Level Household Survey (DLHS) and Youth in India (National Youth Study) were also examined for their SRH component of young people. Information was sorted by year and themes. After screening for eligibility, a total of **277** articles (full texts as well as abstracts) were found in first-level searches, and **191** were finally included in the review.

5.2 SRH of Young People: An Overview

Most studies do not make a distinction between adolescents and youth, i.e. study participants/respondents fall in age group of 15–24, encompassing 15–19-year-old adolescents and 20–24-year-old youth. Further, studies with adult samples considered individuals within 18–30 or 18–45 age group with no segregated data for 18–24, making it difficult to clearly separate these age groups. Most studies based on school children do not mention marital status of participants assuming all would be unmarried though that may not be the case, especially in rural contexts.

Areas of SRH where some research is available include menstruation and menstrual hygiene, early marriage and childbearing, sexual activity, reproductive tract infections (RTIs)/sexually transmitted infections (STIs), human immunodeficiency virus infection/acquired immunodeficiency syndrome (HIV/AIDS), contraceptive use, teenage pregnancy, abortion and sexual abuse and violence. In contrast, research is generally lacking on themes of SRH of people with disabilities, sexual minorities and migrant groups. A brief overview of the information of various SRH indicators along with its source for adolescents and youth in India is presented in Table 5.1.

5.2.1 Menstruation and Menstrual Hygiene

The onset of menstruation is an important physiologic change occurring among girls. Lack of discussion around menstruation leads to young girls not being prepared for it (Garg et al. 2001; Population Council and UNICEF 2013). Menstruation is considered impure and dirty and leads to fear and trauma, with restrictions related to work, sex, food, cooking, household work, exercise, playing, mobility, withdrawal from school and a list of do's and don'ts for girls in India (Garg et al. 2001, 2012;

Table 5.1 Information of various SRH indicators for adolescents and youth in India

		Percentage	Data	Source
Early marriage				
Women married before the age of	15 years	27%	National Family Health Survey-3	IIPS and Macro International, National Family Health Survey (NFHS-3), India Report, 2005–2006
	18 years	58%		
15–19 age group who are currently married	Rural women	33%		
	Urban women	15%		
	Rural men	4%		
	Urban men	1%		
Sexual debut				
Before the age of 15 years	Girls	8%	National Family Health Survey-3	IIPS and Macro International, National Family Health Survey (NFHS-3), India, 2005–2006
	Boys	3%		
Between 15 and 24 age group	Women	10%	National Family Health Survey-3	Parasuraman et al. 2009. A Profile of Youth in India, NFHS-3, India, 2005–2006
	Men	2%		
Premarital sex				
In 15–19 age group	Women	25%	Youth in India: Situation and needs	IIPS and Population Council. 2010. Youth in India: Situation and Needs, 2006–2007
	Men	21%		
Genital infection				
Women seeking care for symptoms of genital infections	Overall	40%	Youth in India: Situation and needs	IIPS and Population Council. 2010. Youth in India: Situation and Needs, 2006–2007
	Urban areas	46%	National Behavioural Surveillance Survey (BSS)	NIMS and NACO. 2008, National Behavioural Surveillance Survey (BSS) 2006; youth (15–24 years)
	Rural areas	40%		
Contraception				
Some form of contraception knowledge in 15–19 age group		94%	National Family Health Survey-3	IIPS and Macro International, National Family Health Survey (NFHS-3), India, 2005–2006
Unmet need of contraception in 15–24 age group		23%		
Violence				
Men reporting perpetrating violence	Physical	19%	Youth in India: Situation and needs	IIPS and Population Council. 2010. Youth in India: Situation and Needs, 2006–2007
	Sexual	6%		

Kamaljit et al. 2012; Population Council and UNICEF 2013; Varghese et al. 2015; Van Eijk et al. 2016; Bachloo et al. 2016; Thakur and Holambe 2016; Hossain and Sen 2017; Rajagopal and Mathur 2017; Upadhyay et al. 2018).

Most girls and women do not receive information regarding menstruation before menarche (Thakur et al. 2014; Nagaraj and Konapur 2016; Mohanty et al. 2016; Kusuma and Ahmed 2016; Rajagopal and Mathur 2017). Overall, one fourth of the girls in India know about the uterus as the source of bleeding, and half of them consider menstruation to be a normal process (Van Eijk et al. 2016); however, such knowledge is high in certain areas (95% in rural Haryana; see Kamaljit et al. 2012; 63% in urban Bhopal; see Sinha and Modi 2014; and 61% in urban Amritsar; see Sharma et al. 2016). Knowledge about menstruation is received from friends or sisters-in-law who are comfortable talking about it (Garg et al. 2001; Thakur et al. 2014). Premenarchal knowledge of urban girls is better than those in rural (Datta et al. 2012). Earlier, mothers were hesitant to talk to their daughters about menstruation (Garg et al. 2001), but recent study in urban areas shows that they are major contributor in providing knowledge (Thakur et al. 2014; Van Eijk et al. 2016; Mohanty et al. 2016; Thakur and Holambe 2016), thus highlighting the changing role of mothers.

Poor menstrual hygiene is a major contributor to RTI and female morbidity (Garg et al. 2012). Evidence on use of various absorbents for menstrual hygiene is mixed, e.g. the use of commercially available sanitary pads ranges between 70% (Kamath et al. 2013) and 12% (Sinha 2011). Most of the adolescent girls in rural areas and urban slums report using old cloth pieces or rags (Garg et al. 2001), making them susceptible to RTIs, if not cleaned and dried regularly (Garg et al. 2012). Use of commercial pad has increased over time (Mohanty et al. 2016; Rajagopal and Mathur 2017); cloth is more commonly used in rural areas (Patil and Udgiri 2016) and reported more in community-based studies as compared to school-based studies. Use of absorbents and sanitary pads shows wide rural-urban differences with higher usage in urban areas as compared to rural (Kamaljit et al. 2012; Sharma et al. 2016; Mudey et al. 2016; Kotian et al. 2017). Good menstrual hygiene is associated with good knowledge of menstruation prior to menarche, usage of proper sanitary latrine at home and exposure to media (Ray and Dasgupta 2012).

A recent systematic review and meta-analysis based on 138 existing Indian studies on menstrual hygiene over the last 15 years (Van Eijk et al. 2016) reports that disposal of absorbents is mainly through garbage bins and burning in urban areas, whereas in rural areas absorbents are thrown away in open spaces or buried, the latter more commonly reported in community-based studies. Some studies report avoidance of bathing due to non-availability of bathing space, lack of privacy, scarcity of water and belief that it would lead to problems in future pregnancy (Van Eijk et al. 2016).

Menstrual irregularity, premenstrual syndrome (PMS), menstrual practices of people with disability and boys' and men's perspective on menstrual health are understudied areas. While in North India, the prevalence of dysmenorrhoea was slightly less than three fourths among school-going girls (Sachan et al. 2012; Sinha et al. 2017), a study in rural Bijapur found it to be 28% (Patil and Angadi 2013).

Many young girls experience menstrual pain (more than 90% of college-going girls in Moradabad, UP), but less than half of them seek any medical treatment for it (Shukla et al. 2016). A facility-based study in Pondicherry showed that 41% of urban girls and 52% of rural girls were suffering from PMS, whereas a community-based study in rural West Bengal reported that 62% girls were experiencing PMS (Sarkar et al. 2016). Girls only seek treatment for it when the symptoms became severe and hampered their daily functioning (Ramya et al. 2014). Adolescent girls with intellectual disability are unable to change their sanitary pads and communicate their physical discomfort to their caretakers (Thapa and Sivakami 2017). In some cases, the caretakers change sanitary pads of the adolescent girls with disability themselves or try training the girls to maintain hygiene, whereas in some cases, the caretakers may get the uterus of the girls surgically removed for cessation of menstruation (Thapa and Sivakami 2017). Most boys have shown limited biological understanding of menstruation, but they are well aware of the customs and taboos surrounding menstruation (Mason et al. 2017). Boys usually received information regarding menstruation either by overhearing conversations or by observing custom rituals (Mason et al. 2017).

5.2.2 Early Marriage and Childbearing

Although legal age at marriage is 18 years for girls and 21 years for boys (MOLJ 2007), child marriage is still prevalent in some parts of India (Sajitha 2017) where it has societal and cultural approval. In NFHS-3, 58% of all women surveyed in the 20–49 age group were married before age 18 and 27% before age 15 (IIPS and Macro International 2007). Half of the women in 15–24 age group and 19% of women in 15–17 age group were currently married; whereas one fifth of the men were currently married in 15–24 age group and 7% of men were married between the age of 15 and 20 years (Parasuraman et al. 2009). In the 15–19 age group, 27% of the girls were currently married, and 15% and 33% of the urban and rural women were married; while 1% urban and 4% rural men were married in the same age group (IIPS and Macro International 2007), thus highlighting a rural-urban and gender difference. Significant differences based on levels of education have been reported. For example, proportion of women aged 15–19 years who have begun childbearing is half in urban areas as compared to rural areas (9% and 19%, respectively). Moreover, more than one fourth of women without education in this age group became mothers (IIPS and Macro International 2007). Age at marriage affects women's autonomy in family planning, contraception use, experience of domestic violence and institutional delivery (Santhya et al. 2010).

A recent qualitative study on understanding reasons for child marriage reported parents' fear and worry over children's transgression of sexuality norms as the main reason. The fear that young boys or girls would bring dishonour to family through their sexual conduct, household need for unpaid labour, poverty, economic instability, death or desertion of father of the girl's family, or calamities such as floods or riots lead to girls being considered as a burden on household, and the offshoots of marriage in the form of dowry and bride price brought some relief to such families. Violence in natal homes and uncontrollable sexual attraction experienced by young people were other reasons for eloping and marrying before age 18 (TISS and UNFPA 2015).

NFHS-3 showed a strong association between years of education, early marriage and absenteeism in schools (Population Council and UNICEF 2013), for example, only 13% of the women who completed at least 10 years of education were married by the age of 18 as opposed to 72% of the women who had no education at all (IIPS and Macro International 2007). Girls with secondary or higher secondary education would marry older as compared to girls with less than 10 years of education (Nanda et al. 2014). Being in school provides no guarantee in delaying marriage, but dropping out of school surely did provide an additional reason for parents to marry their children (Verma et al. 2013).

Early marriage leads to early childbearing (Naroor and Tribuwan 2017) with 12% of women in 15–19 age group already having a child (IIPS and Macro International 2007). After marriage, girls feel pressurised to reproduce and give birth to a male child (TISS and UNFPA 2015). High risk of pregnancy complication owing to physiological immaturity and inexperience associated with child care practices also influences child and maternal health (Population Council and UNICEF 2013). The risk of maternal death is three times higher in 15–19 years and five times in less than 15 years, as compared to women in their twenties (Barua et al. 2007; Population Council and UNICEF 2013); moreover repeated pregnancies, stillbirths, miscarriages and complications during childbirth are consistently reported in adolescent pregnancies (Mukhopadhyay et al. 2010; Santhya et al. 2010; Patidar 2015; TISS and UNFPA 2015; Patra 2016; Naroor and Tribhuwan 2017).

5.2.3 Sexual Activity

Premarital sex among adolescents is gaining attention in most developing countries including India. NFHS-3 data shows 3% of the boys and 8% of the girls report sexual debut before the age of 15 (IIPS and Macro International 2007). In 15–24 age group, sexual initiation among young men was 2% as compared to 10% in women (Parasuraman et al. 2009) which could be due to more girls getting married before the age of 18 (Population Council and UNICEF 2013). Sexual activity reported among unmarried female youth varies between 2% and 5% across various studies (Alexander et al. 2007; Shekhar et al. 2007; Sujay 2009) whereas for male youth from 10% to 18% (Alexander et al. 2007; Shekhar et al. 2007; Parasuraman et al. 2009; Sujay 2009).

About 7% of young men and 0.5% of young women reported having sexual intercourse with more than one partner in the 12 months preceding NFHS-3 (Parasuraman et al. 2009; Population Council and UNICEF 2013). However, the first-ever National Youth Study indicated higher prevalence of premarital sex (21%

of men and 25% of women aged 15–19) and multiple sexual partners (IIPS and Population Council 2010). Rural-urban differences in sexual activities have been found in never-married youth, with proportions being higher for rural as compared to urban. Besides multiple partner sex activity, a significant number of young people report not using condom during sexual intercourse (Parasuraman et al. 2009).

Adolescents studying in vernacular schools, accessing pornography, who hadn't read scientific literature on reproductive and sexual health, who are sexually abused and who did not have a friendly relationship with their parents were more likely to initiate sexual activity early in their life (Sahay et al. 2013). Adolescents who had initiated sex early were found to be more likely to have symptoms of sexually transmitted disease (Sahay et al. 2013). Despite only a few studies on sexual activity, these studies point to the fact that high risk behaviour is prevalent among adolescents and young population in India.

5.2.4 RTIs and STIs

The prevalence of self-reported RTI symptoms has been found to be 11–18% among women in large surveys (Bhanderi and Kannan 2010) and 40–57% in small-scale studies (Sudha et al. 2007). Young married women are more likely to report symptoms of genital infection as compared to unmarried women and men (IIPS and Population Council 2010). In NFHS-3, unmarried men in 15–24 age group are more likely to report RTI/STI symptoms as compared to married men (Parasuraman et al. 2009).

In DLHS-3, only one fourth of married adolescents were aware about symptoms of RTIs and STIs with lesser awareness among rural women and young people in lowest wealth quantiles (Prusty and Unisa 2013). Knowledge about symptoms of RTI was poor among young women (Hegde et al. 2013) and adolescent girls (Mahanta et al. 2016; Jain et al. 2016; Rajpoot and Gupta 2016). Knowledge about symptoms of STIs is low among adolescents (Raut and Pakhare 2016). Adolescent girls showed slightly better knowledge as compared to boys regarding STIs (Nayak et al. 2016). Men are more concerned about avoiding infections and securing sexual pleasure and less concerned about avoiding potential pregnancies; thus, more men are aware about the role of condom in preventing HIV/AIDS as compared to preventing unwanted pregnancy (Char et al. 2011).

Seeking treatment for symptoms related to RTI and STI is low (Sarkar et al. 2013; Chauhan et al. 2016) with more young people seeking treatment in urban areas (46%) as compared to rural areas (40%) (NACO 2008). Only 40% of young women experiencing symptoms of genital infection seek care (IIPS and Population Council 2010) with married adolescent girls and women showing less likeliness towards seeking treatment in some studies (Santhya and Jejeebhoy 2003; Andrew and Patel 2002) whereas unmarried women showing less likeliness in others (Sabarwal and Santhya 2012). Both married and unmarried women prefer to seek treatment in private sector as compared to public sector facility (Sabarwal and Santhya 2012).

5.2.5 HIV/AIDS

Globally, India accounts for about 7% of HIV-infected adolescents in 10–19 age group, with HIV-related mortality accounting for 9% and 11% of 15–19-year-old adolescents being newly infected (Arpadi 2000). Even with national programmes dedicated to reducing HIV/AIDS in India, multiple studies highlight poor knowledge regarding HIV/AIDS (57% of adolescents and young people in Mumbai slums have poor knowledge) (Velhal et al. 2012) and its mode of transmission in urban (Shinde et al. 2017; Verma et al. 2016; McManus and Dhar 2008) as well as rural areas (Yadav et al. 2011; Mahajan and Sharma 2005b).

Among young people, married young women are at distinct risk of HIV due to relative lack of awareness of HIV and safe sex practices, their lower self-perception of risk, lack of agency and unequal gender norms (Santhya and Jejeebhoy 2007b). Young women who engage in commercial sexual activity (either due to economic reasons or coercion) are stigmatised by the society leading to their inability to access information and health services; whereas married young women engaging in sexual activity with multiple partners may not disclose their HIV status to their husbands or families due to fear of desertion or domestic violence and may fail to access health services due to the same (Chakrapani et al. 2009).

Perinatally infected infants, children and adolescents are medically compromised with consequences such as stunting and micronutrient deficiency (Arpadi 2000). The effect of HIV/AIDS is not only limited to those who are infected but also to their family members as the consequences are not only physical but also emotional (Sen 2005; Pandve et al. 2008). Infected children and adolescents or the ones with infected parents face discrimination by their HIV-negative peers who tend to terminate friendship with them or may bully them (Nath 2009). Further, children face a double burden of coping with the illness and sustaining themselves when they acquire the infection from their parents as they begin considering themselves as a victim and develop a tendency to blame themselves (Naswa and Marfatia 2010).

Adolescents might not even know if they are infected, and even if they do, they might not want to disclose their positive status to their families or friends for fear of repercussions such as being bullied, reprimanded, disowned or even stigmatised (Arpadi 2000). They are worst hit when positive parents die due to the illness which leads to being orphaned, many a times homeless, giving rise to child-headed homes, where they might have to take care of their siblings (Meier 2003). Such a scenario requires them to drop out from school, face economic hardships, be a victim of abuse and exploitation, use drugs and get into conflicts with the society and law (Lala 2014). The developmental milestones of children or adolescent infected with HIV get affected by the illness and also by non-HIV factors such as poverty, inadequate medical services and lack of social support (Brown and Lourie 2000).

5.2.6 Contraceptive Use

Knowledge about contraception is low among adolescent girls (Mahanta et al. 2016; Shankar et al. 2017). Around two thirds of the married adolescent girls knew about at least one method of modern reversible contraceptive technique (Pachauri and Santhya 2002). However, NFHS-3 reveals that some form of contraceptive knowledge has increased with 94% among 15–19-year-olds (IIPS and Macro International 2007). There is difference in the level of awareness regarding emergency contraceptive among girls from medical and allied backgrounds and girls from non-medical backgrounds (Shelat et al. 2012). While youth studying in a medical college in Kerala showed above average knowledge (79% knew about the correct time for administering the pill) regarding emergency contraceptives and their usage (Mohammad Iliyas 2016), the adolescent girls from rural Maharashtra showed little awareness (9% from higher socio-economic groups and 2% from lower socio-economic group) regarding emergency contraceptives (Kakani and Jaiswal 2012). While some research showed adolescent girls were aware than boys about oral and emergency contraceptives (Jain et al. 2014), other showed that young men were more aware about the usage of emergency contraceptives (Joseph et al. 2015).

Condom use during last sexual encounter and consistent condom use are low among unmarried adolescents who report premarital sex (Santhya et al. 2011a). Unmet need of contraception is 23% in 15–24 age group (IIPS and Macro International 2007) with a significant unmet need among young women to delay their first pregnancy (Jejeebhoy et al. 2014b). Condoms were the most common contraceptive used followed by oral contraceptives and traditional methods among young women (Jejeebhoy et al. 2014b). More young women report condom use as compared to men and are more likely to report it if the sexual encounter was with a romantic partner as compared to other partner (Santhya et al. 2011a). In Bihar and Jharkhand, contraceptive use was found to be almost similar among unmarried and married young women (Zavier and Jejeebhoy 2015). Hesitation in approaching anyone for obtaining contraceptive, lack of access to the product, perception of not being at risk (Population Council and UNICEF 2013), perception that the partner is 'safe' (Santhya et al. 2011a), lack of awareness and unplanned nature of sex (Alexander et al. 2007) have been cited as some of the reasons for irregular or non-use of condoms.

5.2.7 Teenage Pregnancy

Teenage pregnancy has far-reaching consequence for young women and the children. Low socio-economic status, lack of primary education (Dutta et al. 2014), knowledge about contraception not getting translated into behaviour, cultural factors and extended family structure have been cited as major factors affecting teenage pregnancy (Acharya et al. 2014). Multiple studies show a higher proportion of pregnant adolescent girls are anaemic as opposed to pregnant adult women (Dutta and Joshi 2013; Spandana et al. 2016; Raghav et al. 2013; Kamini and Avvaru 2014;

Tripathi and Sherchand 2014; Nair and Devi 2015; Rao et al. 2017) and encounter more complications during the term as well as during the delivery (Dutta and Joshi 2013; Talawar and Venkatesh 2013; Spandana et al. 2016). Preterm birth (Kamini and Avvaru 2014; Rupakala et al. 2013; Doddihal and Katti 2017; Rao et al. 2017), caesarean section (Mukhopadhyay et al. 2010; Dutta and Joshi 2013), pre-eclampsia (Nair and Devi 2015; Medhi et al. 2016), stillbirths, neonatal deaths and low birth weight babies were seen as outcomes in higher proportion of teenage pregnancies (Kumar et al. 2007; Mukhopadhyay et al. 2010; Rudra et al. 2013; Shrivastav et al. 2016).

5.2.8 *Abortion*

The evidence for abortion-related experiences of unmarried young adolescents and women is sparse (Ganatra 2000). Facility-based studies show a significant proportion of women seeking abortion are unmarried (Ganatra 2000; Trikha 2001; Devi et al. 2007). In Gujrat, 8–12% of sexually experienced young women or girlfriends of young men who were sexually active had unintended pregnancies which were all terminated (Sujay 2009). More than 50% of the adolescent girls are likely to seek services for abortion from an unauthorised facility (Trikha 2001). The main reason cited for abortion was a previous child being too young or to delay the first birth either due to work, studying in college or doing a vocational training course (Ganatra and Hirve 2002; Population Council and UNICEF 2013).

One fourth of the young girls delay seeking abortion into the second trimester (Jejeebhoy et al. 2010). The reasons for delay in abortion care were found to be lack of support from family and society, the cost of care, issues about confidentiality and condemning nature of health providers, single girls being forced to pay higher fees for seeking the services (Ganatra and Hirve 2002), delay in suspecting pregnancy due to existing menstrual irregularities, delay in confirming pregnancy, delay in clinics due to time taken to arrange supplies for abortion and insisting on being accompanied by a female companion for support (Sowmini 2013).

5.2.9 *Sexual Abuse and Violence*

One third of the women have experienced physical or sexual violence in India (IIPS and Population Council 2010). Non-consensual sexual relations amount for 18% and 2% of the current pregnancies among unmarried and married adolescents (Jejeebhoy et al. 2010). While married women in Bihar experienced physical and sexual violence in early days of their marriage (Jejeebhoy et al. 2013), 14% of college-going girls in Gujarat (Sujay 2009), 10% in Andhra Pradesh and 25% in Madhya Pradesh (Santhya et al. 2008) report their first sexual encounter being forced even with romantic partners. In semi-urban area of Najafgarh in Delhi, 27%

of the girls had experienced sexual abuse, and one in ten had experienced severe form of sexual abuse (Daral et al. 2016). The perpetrators of sexual abuse for girls were relatives, friends and neighbours (Daral et al. 2016). Women who made their own decisions and showed self-efficacy were less likely to experience physical and sexual violence (Acharya et al. 2009; IIPS and Population Council 2010). Women in households with high standard of living and who were fairly or very familiar with their husband at the time of their marriage were less likely to experience occasional or frequent unwanted sex (Santhya et al. 2007). Youth study showed that men were more likely to report perpetrating physical violence than sexual violence; 19% reported perpetrating physical violence, but only 6% reported that they had forced their wife to have sexual relations (IIPS and Population Council 2010; Population Council and UNICEF 2013).

5.3 Research Gaps

This section highlights key research gaps in existing studies on the topic. Overall, there seems to be serious lack of evidence for younger adolescents (10–14) and married adolescents (both girls and boys). There is a tendency to treat married adolescents along with married women though the married adolescents have different needs and are much more vulnerable in negotiating with their spouse and other family members on various issues of SRH. The specific gaps are discussed below.

Menstrual hygiene has been mainly studied among 10–15-year-old girls; very few studies look at the practices of 16–18-year-old girls, married adolescent girls and unmarried and married young women. Thus, there is lack of understanding about forms of transition in hygiene practices from adolescent girls to young women. Few studies exist regarding menstrual irregularities such as dysmenorrhoea, oligomenorrhoea, etc. among adolescent girls and young women. Further, rarely studies focus on knowledge of gatekeepers like parents and teachers who can act as agent of change in ensuring better menstrual health. Recognising the importance of delaying childbirth among married adolescents, research is needed on finer context-specific cultural nuances related to early marriage and how they negotiate with their spouse and family members to delay their conception.

Greater exposure to sexual content through electronic media is leading to increased experimentation with sex. Early sexual debut, premarital sexual activity and multiple partners are seen, but the evidence for the factors associated with these is sparse. RTIs/STIs are rarely studied in the age group of 10–14 years for both adolescent boys and girls. Although HIV/AIDS has been researched to a certain extent in the 10–14 age group, the focus is more on the knowledge and very less on behaviour and attitude towards safe sexual practices. There is very little understanding regarding the adolescents who have acquired HIV perinatally, their issues related to disclosure to family, relatives and sexual partners, bereavement, compliance towards medication, side effects of long-term medication, stigma and what it means to live with HIV as an adolescent. Research regarding emergency contraceptives, its knowledge and use among adolescents and youth is required. There should be an inquiry into the factors associated with teenage pregnancy among the unmarried girls from a more sociocultural, economic and geographical understanding rather than the clinical aspect of it. Most studies on sexual activity, contraceptive use and RTI/STI, consider young people from 15–24 years, which treats the entire group as homogeneous and does not take into account their various vulnerabilities such as caste, socio-economic status, gender, marital status, geographic location and so on of each group. This is a serious gap, and hence a segregated data from 10 to 14, 15 to 19 and 20 to 24 would be useful, especially from education and counselling point of view.

Lack of knowledge, premarital sex and unmet need of contraception lead to unwanted pregnancies for which women seek abortion. Due to pre-existing taboos and sensitivity around the issue, the literature on abortion among unmarried girls is less. There is a need to understand experiences of unmarried women seeking abortion and the attitude of health professionals towards them and collect segregated data for adolescent girls and young women. Research on married women seeking abortion, their reasons and decision-making related to abortion is lacking. Issues around sexual violence are much less studied among adolescents in general and unmarried adolescent girls in particular as compared to young women. Among young women (including married), there are very few studies on sexual violence.

Evidence for such issues from life course perspective is required to see how improper menstrual hygiene, early or delayed treatment of RTIs/STIs, teenage pregnancy, abortion and sexual abuse can individually or synergistically affect sexual and reproductive health of women in the future. Studies on multicultural societies and their myriad perceptions about gender roles, early marriage and social hierarchies need to be conducted to understand their effect on sexual and reproductive health of adolescents and youth.

Very few studies exist on masculinity and gender roles in 10–14 age group. It is during this age group, gender roles are acquired and internalised, and hence it is imperative to understand the problem at this level. Studies on masculinity, adolescent boys' perspective about their roles and responsibilities during teenage pregnancy, and young men's vulnerabilities in decision-making and their role in contraceptive use and delaying pregnancy are few. Research on boys and young men about their perceptions of menstruation, boys who have been married early and the challenges they face in living a married life in their adolescence is completely lacking. There is lack of evidence from men's perspective in involvement and decision-making for abortion, men's understanding of women who seek abortion services, and men's perceived reasons for abandoning women who undergo abortion.

There is almost no inquiry to understand why men perpetrate sexual abuse and violence on women and how do gender roles shape such attitude and behaviour among them. There is absolutely no literature to look at sexual abuse and violence on adolescent boys, young men and the lesbian, gay, bisexual and transgender (LGBT) communities. Comparison on the sexual abuse and violence among women, adolescent boys, young men and LGBT communities and their implications on the sexual reproductive health is much needed. More research is needed to understand the role of adolescent boys and young men as gatekeepers of women's sexual and reproductive health.

Practically, there is no study on SRH issues of people with disability (PWDs) in India. Their perceptions, experiences and challenges need to be understood and addressed. There is a tendency to treat them as asexual, and hence even the recognition of their issues in the research area is weak. Studies focusing on alternative sexuality of adolescents and young people are few in India. This needs to be urgently addressed as there is very little information on their experiences.

5.4 Barriers for Young People to Seeking SRH Services

Taboo surrounding SRH coupled with additional vulnerabilities like lack of awareness about the issues, peer influence and dependency on parents/guardian lead to facing barriers in availing health services for SRH among young people. We have tried to look at the barriers faced by young people within the ecological model (Bronfenbrenner 1977) under three headings: (a) individual-level barriers, (b) familial/community-level barriers and (c) systems-level barriers (see Fig. 5.1).

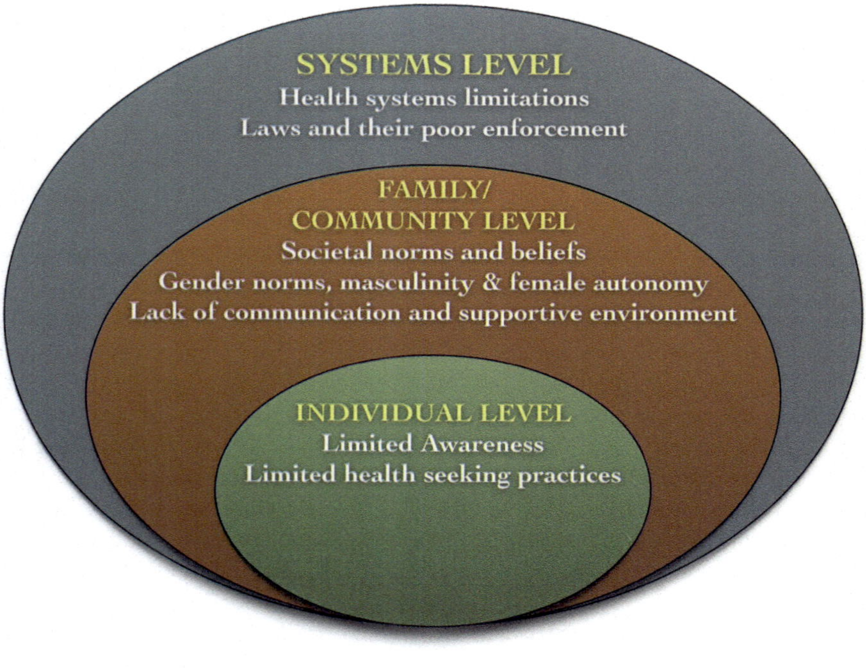

Fig. 5.1 Barriers for seeking sexual and reproductive health among young people

5.4.1 *Individual-Level Barriers*

Women living in rural areas (IIPS and Macro International 2007), with less or no education, belonging to scheduled castes or scheduled tribes and poor households (Santhya and Jejeebhoy 2012), are more likely to have their first birth before the age of 18 years. Knowledge about SRH issues is higher in young people who are educated, from urban areas and from high-income households (MOHFW 2009). Economic status (Kesterton et al. 2010), place of residence, women's education, husbands' education (Singh et al. 2012) and birth order and interval (Parasuraman et al. 2009) are significant determinants for access and utilisation of services.

5.4.1.1 Limited Awareness

Knowledge about menstruation prior to menarche is very little (Mudey et al. 2016), causing fear among young girls at its onset (UNICEF 2012). Awareness regarding maintaining menstrual hygiene is low (UNICEF 2012). Painful menstruation and white discharge were seen as minor inconveniences, and unmarried girls sought advice from their mothers, whereas married women from their husband, rarely from their mother-in-law, for these issues (Barua and Kurz 2001).

Large-scale studies show that knowledge about at least one method of contraception is high (rural and unmarried women have lesser knowledge than others) (IIPS and Population Council 2010), but small-scale studies indicate in-depth understanding of contraceptive method (Acharya et al. 2009; Dorairajan, et al. 2015) and consistent use of it are far from universal (Sujay 2009). Use of contraception is low among unmarried young women due to its limited accessibility to them as compared to married young women (MOHFW 2009). Knowledge regarding legality of abortion for unmarried and married women and illegality of seeking abortion after 20 weeks or termination of female foetus was limited (IIPS and Population Council 2010).

5.4.1.2 Limited Health-Seeking Practices

Adolescents are more likely than young women to seek abortion from unqualified health providers (Santhya and Jejeebhoy 2012). Moreover, unmarried adolescents have been reported to undergo delayed abortion due to cost of care and confidentiality issues (Ganatra and Hirve 2002; Jejeebhoy et al. 2010; Nath and Garg 2008). Delay in recognizing pregnancy, failed attempts to terminate pregnancy, and lack of partner support are additional barriers to seeking abortion services (Jejeebhoy et al. 2010; Population Council and UNICEF 2013).

More young men than women, 56% and 40% respectively, seek treatment for genital infections in the presence of symptoms (IIPS and Population Council 2010). Limited care-seeking for symptoms of gynaecological morbidity has also been observed in other studies (Andrew and Patel 2002; Barua and Kurz 2001; Prasad et al. 2005; Rani and Bonu 2003; Santhya and Jejeebhoy 2012). Facility-based survey in Bhavnagar reveals that only 13% of the girls suffering from RTIs sought treatment and the main reasons for not seeking treatment were shyness, financial constraints and lack of awareness about services (Chauhan et al. 2016).

5.4.2 *Familial/Community-Level Barriers*

5.4.2.1 Lack of Communication and Supportive Environment

While newly-wed adolescent girls are expected to prove their fertility (Barua and Kurz 2001; TISS-UNFPA 2015), the men are expected to establish their 'manliness' by providing a child, thus, compromising the autonomy and negotiating power of newly-wed couples in deciding the timing of their first child (Sethuraman et al. 2007) and limiting healthcare or contraception for adolescent girls, as the decision-makers are either their husband or mother-in-law (Santhya and Jejeebhoy 2003). While some girls approach their mothers about menstrual irregularities or burning urination, mother-in-law is never approached for such problems as it may be seen as a threat to conception (Barua and Kurz 2001).

Adolescent-parent communication on topics such as romantic relationships, reproduction or other SRH issues is very less (Jejeebhoy and Santhya 2011a) for both boys and girls with rural-urban difference, i.e. urban women were more likely to discuss such issues with their mothers as compared to rural (IIPS and Population Council 2010). More than three fourths of the young women had discussed matters of growing up which was limited to mechanics of menstruation and behavioural do's and don'ts (IIPS and Population Council 2010). Better spousal communication on SRH showed greater utilisation of antenatal care and shared decision-making regarding place of delivery (Rani et al. 2007). While most unmarried girls prefer parents to provide family life/sex education than healthcare providers (Tripathi and Sekhar 2013), parents feel embarrassed in discussing sexual topic because either they themselves lack adequate knowledge (Mahajan and Sharma 2005a) or they consider such conversations are inappropriate before marriage, against the existing cultural norms, and would negatively affect child's sexual behaviour and encourage adolescents to engage in sexual activity (Jejeebhoy and Santhya 2011a; Guilamo-Ramos et al. 2012).

5.4.2.2 Gender Norms, Masculinity and Female Autonomy

In India, masculinity is associated with toughness and dominance, sexual potency, absence of feminine characteristics and proving manhood through aggression and sexually coercive behaviour (Verma and Mahendra 2005), whereas femininity is associated with submissiveness and an ideal woman should not respond to men's sexual advances (Verma et al. 2006). Such roles show greater acceptance of violence against women (Das et al. 2014) and contribute to vulnerability of married adolescents and young women to HIV, for example, premarital relations are acceptable for men but not for women (Santhya and Jejeebhoy 2007a; Population Council and UNICEF 2013). Condom use is not a priority among young men as sexual activity may occur in a hurry or in coercion, and girlfriends or wives are not perceived risky (Verma et al. 2006). Sensitisation of men towards gender norms leads to better gender attitudes, behavioural change, lesser physical violence (Achyut et al. 2011), higher condom use and better communication about HIV and STIs (Verma et al. 2008; Das et al. 2014).

Decision-making autonomy and freedom of movement are higher among young women (20–24 years) living in urban areas, from higher caste, more educated and wealthier households (IIPS and Population Council 2010; Santhya and Jejeebhoy 2012). Women's autonomy has been linked to utilisation of antenatal care services (Rani et al. 2007). Limited agency in decision-making (Santhya and Jejeebhoy 2012), freedom of mobility (Nath and Garg 2008), self-efficacy and financial resources (Banerjee et al. 2015) are the factors which limit their access to information on SRH and seeking health services (MOHFW 2009). Parents for unmarried women and husbands for married woman have been the decision-makers for seeking abortion services (Jejeebhoy et al. 2010). Married adolescent girls have lesser social support, social networks and restricted mobility (Mathur et al. 2003). The National Youth Study showed that most men and women believed that a woman should obtain her husband's permission for most things and more than half of them agreed that wife beating was justified if a woman disagrees with her husband's opinion, goes out without telling her husband, is unfaithful or refuses sex (IIPS and Population Council 2010).

5.4.2.3 Societal Norms and Beliefs

The societal norms create taboos around premarital relationships leading to less reporting (Collumbein et al. 2011) in not only community-based surveys by both men and women (IIPS and Population Council 2010) but also large-scale studies like NFHS (Population Council and UNICEF 2013), and thus contributing to barrier in meeting needs of young people. Cultural beliefs in society lead to more psychosexual problems like anxiety among men regarding semen loss and semen weakness (Collumbein and Hawkes 2000). Men feel uncomfortable or embarrassed to access condom due to cultural norms that prevent them from indulging in such behaviour (Char et al. 2011). Women with symptoms of RTIs express guilt and shame due to perceived association of RTIs with sexual infidelity, thus delaying treatment (Barua and Kurz 2001; Prasad et al. 2005). Muslim women are less likely to seek institutional delivery compared to Hindu women (Navaneetham and Dharmalingam 2002), and the 'purdah' system requiring them to cover their bodies has been found to be factor for such low utilisation of services (Hazarika 2011).

5.4.3 Systems-Level Barriers

5.4.3.1 Health System Limitations

The high unmet need of contraception could be due to supply-side hurdles and inability of family planning programme to cater to special needs of young women (Parasuraman et al. 2009). The Adolescent Education Programme (AEP) was launched in 1993, but there is no consensus among state governments leading to many states not including sex education in the curriculum (Population Council and UNICEF 2013). Although teachers have shown a favourable attitude towards sex education, they have also reported that they require special training to discuss sexuality with adolescents (Toor 2012). There is unmet need of family life/sex education (FLE) among unmarried young women (Dorairajan et al. 2015), and women from lower wealth quantiles have much less exposure to FLE (Tripathi and Sekhar 2013). Most programmes focus on in-school adolescents excluding the marginalised who are mostly out of school, and the programmes which focus on out-of-school adolescents end up addressing more boys than girls (Santhya and Jejeebhoy 2012).

Abortion services are rarely available in rural areas (Kalyanwala et al. 2010). Beliefs such as abortion is morally wrong, woman do not always have the right to seek abortion for an unwanted pregnancy and a woman needs to have a partner while seeking abortion (Sjostrom et al. 2014) lead to judgemental (Ganatra and Hirve 2002) and insensitive (CORT 2009) attitudes among providers which act as barrier to women seeking abortion services. Young unmarried men in rural areas feel ignored by health professionals and expect information regarding SRH from them through interpersonal communication (Char et al. 2011). Counsellors have been found to have more gender-balanced clientèle; accredited social health activist (ASHA) and auxiliary nurse midwife (ANM) serve more girls than boys and more married than unmarried; whereas medical officers (MOs) who are men serve more boys than girls and tend to refer girls to female MOs, ASHAs or ANMs (Jejeebhoy et al. 2014a).

Absence of healthcare providers at the facility (Nath and Garg 2008), lack of confidentiality, inadequate quality of care and hesitation in accessing services, in government facilities, have been cited as reasons for visiting private facilities (CORT 2009; Prusty and Unisa 2013). Evaluation of Adolescent Reproductive and Sexual Health (ARSH) strategy suggests that neither services have increased for adolescents nor the quality of services have improved (Santhya and Jejeebhoy 2012). Knowledge about ARSH services is poor, and young people in rural areas and boys are much less aware (CORT 2009; Gupta et al. 2015). Only 7% of young men and 3% of young women received information on sexual matters by healthcare providers (IIPS and Population Council 2010). Training of providers in ARSH clinics is inadequate (CORT 2009) and does not combine the information to be imparted and ways in which it could be imparted (Santhya and Jejeebhoy 2012). ANMs being unable to devote time for counselling due to multiple responsibilities, MOs being overburdened, and shortage of staff are barriers to providing service to adolescents and youth (Jejeebhoy et al. 2014a).

Programmes like Kishori Shakti Yojana (KSY), the SABLA scheme or the University Talk AIDS Programme have not been evaluated yet to assess their effectiveness and acceptability (Santhya and Jejeebhoy 2012). Only 21% adolescents in 15–19 age group received information through interpersonal communication, Chhattisgarh and Madhya Pradesh being at 6% (NACO 2008).

5.4.3.2 Laws and Their Poor Enforcement

Laws such as the Child Marriage Restraint Act, Dowry Prevention Act, Sexual Harassment Act, Preconception and Prenatal Diagnostics Techniques Act and Sexual Harassment at Workplace Bill are in place to promote and ensure positive SRH outcomes among the young, but these laws are poorly implemented which is a major barrier (TISS and UNFPA 2015; Population Council and UNICEF 2013), for example, continuation of marriage of girls and boys under the age of 18 years (TISS and UNFPA 2015). The definition of 'child' is different in different laws which creates loopholes and hampers proper functioning and implementation of the laws. Young girls as well as community at large are not aware of the laws that protect them and promote the sexual and reproductive health of young people (IIPS and Macro International 2007; IIPS and Population Council 2010; Population Council and UNICEF 2013). There is limited evidence about implementation of other acts, and even though efforts are made to increase awareness about them, they are not well documented.

5.5 Challenges in Conducting Research

Conducting research and gathering information from adolescents and young on SRH issues comes with a lot of challenges. In order to understand such challenges, consultation interviews were carried out with key informants (prominent researchers, programme implementers, policy-makers working in civil society organisations and government organisations) in the areas of SRH of adolescents and young people. Interviews were audio recorded and most of them lasted around 40–45 min. Themes explored included challenges experienced by researchers in conducting research on young people within the domain of SRH, samples included and excluded and challenges in conducting large surveys on SRH of adolescents and young people.

Considering young population as a homogeneous group was reiterated as a major challenge in conducting research. Researchers may fail to understand the heterogeneity that exists due to different socio-economic background, age groups, gender, geographical location and marital status within this group. There is vast difference in the needs and issues of young and old, educated and uneducated, urban and rural adolescents and youth due to difference in their level of knowledge and understanding of SRH issues. Obtaining information about issues such as sex from young adolescents is very difficult due to the sensitivity of the issues and their understanding of those. Asking questions in a way which is easily comprehensible, using local terms, is crucial. Getting married adolescents to talk about their issues was identified as a big challenge as they are more socially isolated, under control of in-laws and spouse, and thus the least empowered. Hence, how to reach them, especially for SRH-related themes, is a big question for researchers. There are gender differences within research as well as a lot more focus in SRH research has been on girls and much less data is available on boys.

SRH encompasses myriad sensitive areas – sexual abuse and violence, premarital sex, miscarriage abortion, etc. – and studying these among young people is even more sensitive leading to ethical challenges. Ensuring 'do no harm' becomes a challenge due to the nature of the issues; thus, such areas remain less researched. Maintaining confidentiality regarding the issue is important although the condition would be considered severe by the investigator, for example, the adolescent being interviewed is HIV positive; his/her privacy has to be respected. Mechanisms to provide proper referrals and services to participants of study were also identified as a challenge. Getting consent was found to be another major challenge although some participants didn't feel so. Being clear and communicating about the type of study being conducted, but not getting into detailed description of the questions as parents may feel awkward either due to sensitive nature of questions or may consider it inappropriate for their adolescent children and lose confidence in the researcher, was suggested to ensure more consent and less barrier from the gatekeepers in conducting research (e.g. for a study on premarital sexual activity, parents being informed that we wish to conduct a study on boy-girl relations instead of informing that we need to know about sexual activity of boys and girls).

Different ways of collecting data have been advocated to collect information about sensitive issues. Information about sensitive issues can be collected at the end of the interview because by then there is better rapport and better chances of collecting correct information. For example, in a study on abortion, adolescents seeking services were not asked about their marital status but given the option of declaring it on a piece of paper with the assurance that the information would be accessed only by principal investigator. In another example, in situations where an adolescent is surrounded by other members and not given full privacy, having an extra set of investigators could be helpful to divert other household members with different set of questions, to ensure privacy.

Ensuring quality of data in large-scale studies is another challenge. Interviewer's skills in asking questions are important; hence, training the field researchers, who may belong to the same society and hence have inhibitions in asking questions of sensitive nature to adolescents, was emphasised in order to collect genuine data. Rapport building and asking questions in a way it is sensitive to the respondents were suggested to reduce under-reporting. Some emphasised on the need for the principal investigator to be fully aware and available 24 h to attend to issues or emergencies in the field. Use of clinical measures to improve data quality was considered a valid but expensive method. Though clinical measures were acknowledged to give better estimates, it posed challenge in matching clinical findings with self-reported ones; moreover self-reporting was considered reliable as it focussed on the individual than the laboratory findings.

In longitudinal studies, keeping track of respondents is a challenge as this is a mobile group, migrating to cities, towns or villages due to marriage, for education or for economic pursuits. Age-related changes would increase or decrease vulnerabilities to different conditions. Longitudinal studies need to be started earlier to allow more follow-ups. Monitoring and evaluation by making field visits and attending training and interview sessions to ensure reliable data is needed. What measures should be used to evaluate the outcomes of the programmes poses a challenge. The challenge related to what to measure and how to measure leads to much less evaluation of such programmes and thus less research in these areas.

5.6 Policies for SRH of Young People

The National Population Policy (NPP) 2000 acknowledged young people as underserved group with special SRH needs and advocated strengthening of primary health centres (PHCs) to ensure access to affordable services (MOHFW 2000). The National Health Policy (NHP) 2002 recognised the need to raise awareness and health-promoting behaviour among school- and college-going students (MOHFW 2002a). The National AIDS Prevention and Control Policy (NAPCP) 2002 advocated promoting better understanding of HIV and safe sex practices through enabling environment, and HIV/AIDS education in educational institutions and youth organisations (NACO 2002). The National Youth Policy (NYP) 2003 underscored differential needs of adolescents (13–19 years) and young people (20–35 years) and suggested 'adolescent clinics' and 'youth health associations' for a holistic approach to address their issues (MOYAS 2003). The National Plan of Action for Children (NPAC) 2005 argues for action to build awareness and enable adolescents to access services for SRH (MOWCD 2005). NYP 2014 acknowledged that young people are not a homogeneous group and focuses on creating awareness about SRH issues (especially in rural areas) and providing incentive to health workers for working in rural areas (MOYAS 2014). NHP 2017 puts special emphasis on health challenges of young people, envisages school health programme as a major focus to improve health and hygiene, and aims to expand scope of SRH to address issues like nutrition status, psychological problems linked with misuse of technology, etc. (MOHFW 2017).

5.6.1 Gaps in Policies

NPP 2000 focused on less controversial aspects of SRH and targeted adolescents on counselling and providing information rather than legal and abortion services. It lacked clarity about including unmarried adolescents as most provisions were mainly for married adolescents (Jejeebhoy and Santhya 2011b). NAPCP 2002 failed to mention any special packaged services for young people, focused on unmarried young people and tried to reach out-of-school youth but ended up focusing more on men; thus, married adolescent girls and young women are left out. NHP 2002 does not discuss SRH services and counselling for young people exclusively (Jejeebhoy and Santhya 2011b). NYP 2003 has ambiguity in the kind of services recommended and the extent to which unmarried and girls would be covered, and the 'youth health associations' lack clear strategies to involve more girls and young women (Jejeebhoy and Santhya 2011b). NPP 2000, NAPCP 2002 and NYP 2003 consider young people as a homogeneous group and are vague in operationalising their commitments, rarely describing measures that need to be taken to achieve the goals. NYP 2014 is ambiguous regarding sex education in educational institutions, aims at mainstreaming marginalised group but only in livelihood and not in health and overall lacks a holistic approach towards SRH. NHP 2017 remains silent on the status of FLE and the measures needed to promote it. Further, while it aims to broaden the scope of SRH, it fails to clearly emphasise on areas within SRH which have not been addressed so far.

5.7 Programmes for SRH of Young People

Rashtriya Kishor Swasthya Karyakram (RKSK) 2014 (launched in 231 districts in first phase) aimed to strengthen the adolescent component of the Reproductive Maternal Neonatal Child and Adolescent Health (RMNCH+A) programme. Facility-based services include adolescent-friendly health clinics (AFHC) where clients are registered and provided services and counselling while maintaining confidentiality, and community-based services include peer educators (to some extent ASHAs and ANMs) working with in-school and out-of-school adolescents by forming health clubs, celebrating adolescent health day and sustaining peer education (MOHFW 2014a, b).

Adolescence Education Programme launched by the Ministry of Human Resource Development and National AIDS Control Organisation in 2005 is implemented by the State Council of Educational Research and Training/state boards with the support of State AIDS Control Societies with a focus on providing accurate, culturally relevant information and promoting healthy attitudes regarding SRH through school curriculum (MOHRD 2005; NACO 2008). It is also being implemented at national-level agencies such as Central Board of Secondary Education (CBSE), through the United Nations Population Fund (UNFPA), and civil society organisation in partnership with state education departments (Jaya and Yadav 2010; NCERT 2011).

Adolescent Reproductive and Sexual Health (ARSH) strategy advocates strengthening of existing public health system, creates enabling environment, improves accessibility and provides preventive, promotive, curative and referral services to young people. It recognises special needs of out-of-school youth and aims to raise awareness regarding delaying marriage and first pregnancy, sexual risk-reduction strategies, gender relations and the role of men through ANMs, ASHAs and male health workers (MOHFW 2006).

Red Ribbon Club (RRC) was established under the National AIDS Control Project (II and III) to provide youth-oriented counselling, life skills education, recreation activities and guidance with special focus on districts with high-risk groups or HIV prevalence and was later established for adolescent girls as well with support from the Ministry of Women and Child Development (MWCD) (Jejeebhoy and Santhya 2011b). The University Talk AIDS Programme was to spread awareness of HIV and safe sex among college students (NACO 2004).

School Health Programme was launched under National Rural Health Mission (NRHM) to raise awareness of health, hygiene, nutrition and SRH through curricular and co-curricular approaches (MOHFW 2008). Menstrual Hygiene Scheme under NRHM targets rural adolescents (10–19 years) to improve menstrual hygiene management (MOHFW 2016). Rajiv Gandhi Scheme for Empowerment of Adolescent Girls (RGSEAG)-SABLA, launched by MWCD, replaced KSY and added promoting awareness about ARSH component into it (MOWCD 2010).

Prerna scheme by National Population Stabilisation Fund (functioning in all Empowered Action Group (EAG) states except Uttaranchal) provides monetary incentives to couples who get married after the age of 19, have a child 2 years after marriage, and any one partner choosing permanent method of family planning (Jansankhya Sthirta Kosh 2013). Mamta Taruni Abhiyan in Gujrat provides healthcare to out-of-school adolescent girls (10–19 years) through female health workers, ASHAs and peer educators (CHETNA 2013). Shuchi Yojane in Karnataka promotes menstrual hygiene management through Anganwadi workers (AWW) among in-school and out-of-school adolescent girls regardless of their marital status (Government of Karnataka 2014). Meena Raju Manch Programme in Maharashtra addresses inequitable gender attitudes by promoting awareness among adolescents about their rights, understanding about adolescent development, school sanitation, hygiene and safe drinking water, development of life skills and leadership skills, and promotes the idea of marriage at appropriate age (CORO 2015).

5.7.1 Gaps in Existing Programmes

Implementation of programmes has faced huge obstacles. Implementation of programmes like Janani Suraksha Yojana (JSY) has been uneven with lesser women under 18 years availing its benefits (Lim et al. 2010; Santhya et al. 2011b), whereas counselling of newly married by ASHAs isn't holistic but limited to contraception (Santhya et al. 2011b). The programmes tend to focus on school- and college-going young people; the ones which focus on in-school and out-of-school (MHS, RKSK, SABLA) are designed in the context of rural areas and to a lesser extent for urban areas (Muralidharan et al. 2015).

RKSK acknowledges discrimination faced by adolescents due to their sexual orientation but fails to consider it while formulating strategies with no mention of alternative sexualities in counselling services. In RKSK, it is imperative to know the selection criteria for peer educators, how many peer educators have been engaged, quality of training, their capacity in involving young people in group activities, and what impact has it had on attitudes and behaviour of adolescents living in areas where it is implemented as compared to ones where it isn't for proper monitoring of the programme.

AEP received a political backlash due to its content due to which its implementation is still uneven (Jejeebhoy and Santhya 2011b). Significant efforts were taken to make the content more holistic (NACO 2008), the misconceptions such as marriage ensures safety from infections have not been addressed, and the discussion on contraception is very limited with methods being explained in abstract manner without mentioning pros and cons (Jejeebhoy and Santhya 2011b). The manner in which the SRH component is taught and the competency of teachers who teach these issues are not well known. A comprehensive outlook towards educating gatekeepers as well about SRH is lacking. Periodic quality assessment has shown to improve the quality and utilisation of ARSH clinics, but the community outreach activities have been challenging (Chauhan et al. 2018). Raising awareness under ARSH strategy has been poor as the states have failed to make concerted efforts towards behaviour change communication (MOHFW 2009).

The quality of training imparted to trainers is of concern as young men and women have reported feeling embarrassed and uncomfortable while receiving FLE and inability to clarify doubts (IIPS and Population Council 2010). The funds allocated for training of ASHAs under MHS are much less, thus affecting the quality of training (Muralidharan et al. 2015). The monitoring and evaluation of school-based programmes is weak. The extent of coverage, training, number of students exposed to information, quality and effectiveness of programmes is not known.

5.8 Laws Affecting SRH of Young People

The Child Marriage Restraint Act of 1929 and the Child Marriage Restraint Act of 1978 prohibit marriage to a girl and a boy before reaching age 18 and 21 years, respectively. The Prohibition of Child Marriage Act 2006 is more recent and strengthens the legislation with additional punitive measures and appointment of a Child Marriage Prohibition officer whose task is to prevent such marriages, sensitise communities and collect evidence for effective prosecution of those contravening the provisions of the act (MOLJ 2007). The Protection of Women from Domestic Violence Act 2005 strengthens women's options by adopting a broad definition of domestic violence including actual abuse and threat to abuse, and offers considerable protection, legal aid, healthcare, and economic support (MOWCD 2006). The Prevention of Children from Sexual Offences (POCSO) 2012 seeks to protect children from sexual assault, sexual harassment, prostitution and pornography and provides guidelines for media to sensitively and discreetly report cases of sexual offence and for the establishment of special courts for the trial of such offences

(MOWCD 2013). The MTP Act of 1971 and the 2002 amendments have ensured women's rights to terminate unwanted pregnancy (up to 20 weeks) safely and confidentially irrespective of their marital status and parental consent (GOI 1971; MOHFW 2002b).

5.8.1 Gaps in Existing Laws

There is lack of awareness regarding laws addressing SRH of young people (Ramesh et al. 2016; Kansal et al. 2017), for example, 40% of young women and 30% of young men being unaware about the legal minimum age for marriage (IIPS and Population Council 2010). Young people's awareness about their rights under MTP Act (IIPS and Population Council 2010; Jejeebhoy and Santhya 2011b) and Protection of Women from Domestic Violence Act 2005 is limited due to failure in translation of the act in regional languages and no efforts taken for education and communication to create awareness (Planning Commission 2011).

Prohibition of Child Marriage Act 2006 does not make the registration of marriages compulsory. It neither prohibits child bride from living with her husband nor protects her from sexual or other forms of abuse; moreover, it puts the onus of declaring such a marriage void on the child or the guardians, who would have to go through court proceedings which are serious limitations in its provisioning (Law Commission of India 2008; Jejeebhoy and Santhya 2011b).

Under POCSO Act, mandatory reporting (by everyone including those who may have acquired that information during delivering their professional duty like doctors or counsellors; or within a confidentiality agreement like researchers) of cases of child sexual abuse to law enforcement agencies with information about child's name, age, address, nature of abuse and suspected perpetrator of abuse would lead to cases not coming forward and may make the child vulnerable to more abuse if she/he wishes to report it.

Concerns have also been raised about the different definitions of 'child' in various laws, for example, the Child Marriage Restraint Act (1929 and 1978) defines a child as a male under 21 and a female under 18; Immoral Traffic (Prevention) Act of 1986 defines a child as below 16 years, and a minor between 16 and 18; Juvenile Justice (Care and Protection of Children) Act 2000 defines a child as an individual below 18 years (Law Commission of India 2008).

5.9 Recommendations

Based on the synthesis of literature, the following recommendations are made which can guide future work on SRH of adolescents and young people.

The research on SRH issues of adolescents and youth is marred with gaps in the form of lack of sex- and age-segregated data, and lack of studies on boys regarding most SRH issues and their attitudes towards masculinity and gender roles, younger adolescents, menstrual irregularities, menstrual hygiene transition, emergency contraceptives, teenage pregnancies, decision-making in contraceptive use and abortions, sexual violence within and outside marriage, SRH issues of people with disability and alternative sexuality.

Emerging areas such as urban poor (due to increased urbanisation and migration) and impact of media and information technology may add to the vulnerabilities of adolescents and youth. While some evidence exists, there is a need for more evidence and programmatic action towards these groups to address their vulnerability.

Looking at SRH through multiple perspectives and understanding its multiple complex linkages (e.g. complex linkages between SRH and mental health) is essential. There should be more qualitative research to gain understanding of the lives of the young people with their lived realities, and longitudinal studies to understand the various transitions of the population; which can guide programmes and policies.

Existing government programmes and intervention models by non-governmental organisation (NGOs) on SRH of young people need to be evaluated based on coverage (programmes may not focus as effectively on out-of-school young people), the training of service providers, sensitisation processes, quality of care provided, increasing young people's agency and levels of knowledge on SRH matters; and the findings should be used to strengthen these programmes to ensure that they reach even the most vulnerable groups.

The programmes should not only focus on educating young people about their sexual and reproductive health but also about the existing laws by the constitution which can protect them from abuse or discriminatory treatment by peers or healthcare providers while seeking SRH services.

References

Acharya, R., Kalyanwala, S., Jejeebhoy, S. J., et al. (2009). *Broadening girls' horizons: Effects of a life skills education programme in rural UP*. New Delhi: Population Council.

Acharya, D. R., Bhattarai, R., Poobalan, A., Teijlingen, V. E., & Chapman, G. (2014). Factors associated with teenage pregnancy in South Asia. *Health Science Journal, 4*(1), 3–14.

Achyut, P., Bhatia, N., Singh, A. K., Verma, R. K., Khandekar, S., Pallav, P., & Gaikward, R. (2011). *Building support for gender equality among young adolescents in school: Findings from Mumbai India.* Retrieved from United Nations Girls Education Initiative website http://www.ungei.org/resources/files/GEMS_Building_Support_for_Gender_Equality_Adolescents.pdf. Accessed on 28 Sept 2016.

Alexander, M., Garda, L., Kanade, S., Jejeebhoy, S., & Ganatra, B. (2007). Correlates of premarital relationships among unmarried youth in Pune district, Maharashtra, India. *International Family Planning Perspectives, 33*(4), 150–159.

Andrew, G., & Patel, V. (2002). Health needs of adolescents: A study of health needs of adolescents in higher secondary schools in Goa. *Alto-Porvorim, India: Resource Centre for Adolescent and Child Health.*

Arpadi, S. M. (2000). Growth failure in children with HIV infection. *Journal of Acquired Immune Deficiency Syndromes, 25*(suppl.1), S37–S42.

Bachloo, T., Kumar, R., Goyal, A., Singh, P., Yadav, S. S., Bhardwaj, A., & Mittal, A. (2016). A study on perception and practice of menstruation among school going adolescent girls in district Ambala Haryana, India. *International Journal of Community Medicine And Public Health, 3*(4), 931–937.

Banerjee, S. K., Andersen, K. L., Warvadekar, J., Aich, P., Rawat, A., & Upadhyay, B. (2015). How prepared are young, rural women in India to address their sexual and reproductive health needs? A cross-sectional assessment of youth in Jharkhand. *Reproductive Health, 12*(1), 97–107.

Barua, A., & Kurz, K. (2001). Reproductive health-seeking by married adolescent girls in Maharashtra, India. *Reproductive Health Matters, 9*(17), 53–62.

Barua, A., Apte, H., & Kumar, P. (2007). Care and support of unmarried adolescent girls in Rajasthan. *Economic and Political Weekly, 42*(44), 54–62.

Bhanderi, M. N., & Kannan, S. (2010). Untreated reproductive morbidities among ever married women of slums of Rajkot city, Gujarat: The role of class, distance, provider attitudes, and perceived quality of care. *Journal of Urban Health, 87*(2), 254–263.

Bronfenbrenner, U. (1977). Toward an experimental ecology of human development. *American Psychologist, 32*(7), 513–531.

Brown, L. K., & Lourie, K. J. (2000). Children and adolescents living with HIV and AIDS: A review. *The Journal of Child Psychology and Psychiatry and Allied Disciplines, 41*(1), 81–96.

Center for Operations Research and Training (CORT). (2009). *Assessment of adolescent reproductive and sexual health (ARSH) centers in Gujarat – A report*. Vadodara: CORT.

Chakrapani, V., Newman, P. A., Shunmugam, M., Kurian, A. K., & Dubrow, R. (2009). Barriers to free antiretroviral treatment access for female sex workers in Chennai, India. *AIDS Patient Care and STDs, 23*(11), 973–980.

Char, A., Saavala, M., & Kulmala, T. (2011). Assessing young unmarried men's access to reproductive health information and services in rural India. *BMC Public Health, 11*(1), 476–486.

Chauhan, M. G., Patel, H., & Solanki, H. (2016). Reproductive health problems and treatment seeking behavior among adolescent girls of UHTC field practice area, Govt. Medical College, Bhavnagar. *National Journal of Community Medicine, 7*(5), 355–358.

Chauhan, S. L., Joshi, B. N., Raina, N., & Kulkarni, R. N. (2018). Utilization of quality assessments in improving adolescent reproductive and sexual health services in rural block of Maharashtra, India. *International Journal of Community Medicine And Public Health, 5*(4), 1639–1646.

CHETNA. (2013). *Making health and nutritional information and services accessible to adolescents in the state of Gujrat, India.* Retrieved from CHETNA India website http://chetnaindia.org/wp-content/uploads/2011/12/Moving-Ahead.pdf. Accessed on 2 Oct 2016.

Collumbien, M., & Hawkes, S. (2000). Missing men's messages: Does the reproductive health approach respond to men's sexual health needs? *Culture, Health & Sexuality, 2*(2), 135–150.

Collumbien, M., Mishra, M., & Blackmore, C. (2011). Youth-friendly services in two rural districts of West Bengal and Jharkhand, India: Definite progress, a long way to go. *Reproductive Health Matters, 19*(37), 174–183.

Committee of Resource Organisations (CORO). (2015). *CORO annual report 2014–15*. Retrieved from CORO India website http://coroindia.org/content/resources/Annual_Report_CORO_2014-15.pdf. Accessed on 1 Oct 2016.

Daral, S., Khokhar, A., & Pradhan, S. (2016). Prevalence and determinants of child maltreatment among school-going adolescent girls in a semi-urban area of Delhi, India. *Journal of Tropical Pediatrics, 62*(3), 227–240.

Das, M., Ghosh, S., Verma, R., O'Connor, B., Fewer, S., Virata, M. C., & Miller, E. (2014). Gender attitudes and violence among urban adolescent boys in India. *International Journal of Adolescence and Youth, 19*(1), 99–112.

Datta, A., Manna, N., Datta, M., Sarkar, J., Baur, B., & Datta, S. (2012). Menstruation and menstrual hygiene among adolescent girls of West Bengal, India: A school based comparative study. *Global Journal of Medicine, 1*(5), 50–57.

Devi, I. T., Akoijam, B. S., Nabakishore, N., Jitendra, N., & Nonibala, T. (2007). Characteristics of primigravid women seeking abortion services at a referral center, Manipur. *Indian Journal of Community Medicine, 32*(3), 175–177.

Doddihal, C. R., & Katti, S. M. (2017). A prospective study of adolescent pregnancy complications in a rural area of South India. *International Journal of Research in Medical Sciences, 5*(9), 3939–3942.

Dorairajan, G., Chinnakali, P., & Mohan, B. (2015). Knowledge, attitude & factors affecting potential use of emergency contraception in college students in Puducherry, South India. *The Indian Journal of Medical Research, 141*(1), 122–124.

Dutta, I., & Joshi, P. (2013). Maternal and perinatal outcome in teenage vs. Vicenarian primigravidae-a clinical study. *Journal of Clinical and Diagnostic Research, 7*(12), 2881–2884.

Dutta, I., Jha, N., & Dutta, D. K. (2014). Teenage pregnancy – A socio-demographic study at a rural medical college hospital in Southern India. *Asian Journal of Medical Sciences, 5*(4), 29–33.

Ganatra, B. (2000). Abortion research in India: What we know and what we need to know. In R. Ramasubban & S. J. Jejeebhoy (Eds.), *Women's reproductive health in India*. Jaipur: Rawat Publications.

Ganatra, B., & Hirve, S. (2002). Induced abortions among adolescent women in rural Maharashtra, India. *Reproductive Health Matters, 10*(19), 76–85.

Garg, S., Sharma, N., & Sahay, R. (2001). Socio-cultural aspects of menstruation in an urban slum in Delhi, India. *Reproductive Health Matters, 9*(17), 16–25.

Garg, R., Goyal, S., & Gupta, S. (2012). India moves towards menstrual hygiene: Subsidized sanitary napkins for rural adolescent girls—Issues and challenges. *Maternal and Child Health Journal, 16*(4), 767–774.

General Assembly resolution 70/1, Transforming our world: The 2030 agenda for sustainable development (25 September 2015), available from UN website http://undocs.org/A/RES/70/1

Government of India (GOI). (1971). *The medical termination of pregnancy act (Act. No. 34)*. New Delhi: Government of India.

Government of Karnataka. (2014). *Operational guidelines for "SHUCHI YOJANE"*. Bangalore: Directorate of Health and Family Welfare Services, Government of Karnataka.

Guilamo-Ramos, V., Soletti, A. B., Burnette, D., Sharma, S., Leavitt, S., & McCarthy, K. (2012). Parent–adolescent communication about sex in rural India. US–India collaboration to prevent adolescent HIV. *Qualitative Health Research, 22*(6), 788–800.

Gupta, M., Bhatnagar, N., & Bahugana, P. (2015). Inequity in awareness and utilization of adolescent reproductive and sexual health services in union territory, Chandigarh, North India. *Indian Journal of Public Health, 59*(1), 9–17.

Hazarika, I. (2011). Factors that determine the use of skilled care during delivery in India: Implications for achievement of MDG-5 targets. *Maternal and Child Health Journal, 15*(8), 1381–1388.

Hegde, S. K., Agrawal, T., Ramesh, N., Sugara, M., Joseph, P. M., Singh, S., & Thimmaiah, S. (2013). Reproductive tract infections among women in a peri-urban under privileged area in Bangalore, India: Knowledge, prevalence, and treatment seeking behavior. *Annals of Tropical Medicine and Public Health, 6*(2), 215–220.

Hossain, S., & Sen, V. (2017). Socio cultural taboos and restrictions during menstruation followed by school going adolescent girls in a semi urban area of Jaipur, Rajasthan. *Journal of Pharmacy Practice and Community Medicine, 3*(4), 285–287.

International Institute for Population Sciences (IIPS) and Macro International. (2007). *National family health survey (NFHS-3), India, 2005–06*. Mumbai: IIPS.

International Institute for Population Sciences (IIPS) and Population Council. (2010). *Youth in India: Situation and needs 2006–2007*. Mumbai: IIPS.

Jain, M., Jain, S., Patil, S., & Bang, A. (2014). A study on knowledge attitude and practice of contraception in school going children in Wardha district in Central India. *International Journal of Reproduction, Contraception, Obstetrics and Gynecology, 3*(4), 903–908.

Jain, M. A., Jain, S. M., Patil, S., & Bang, A. (2016). A study on knowledge, attitude and practice of sexually transmitted diseases and HIV in adolescent population in Wardha, Maharashtra, India. *International Journal of Contemporary Pediatrics, 3*(2), 367–372.

Jansankhya Sthirta Kosh. (2013). *Scheme: Prerna strategy*. Retrieved from Jansankhya Sthirta Kosh website http://www.jsk.gov.in/prernastrategy.pdf. Accessed on 2 Oct 2016.

Jaya, J., & Yadav, S. (2010). *Adolescence education programme: Evolution, implementation status and lessons learned*. Paper presented at the second UNFPA Regional workshop on programming for young people: The framework for action, Kathmandu, Nepal.

Jejeebhoy, S. J., & Santhya, K. G. (2011a). *Parent-child communication on sexual and reproductive health matters: Perspectives of mothers and fathers of youth in India*. New Delhi: Population Council.

Jejeebhoy, S. J., & Santhya, K. G. (2011b). *Sexual and reproductive health of young people in India: A review of policies, laws and programs*. New Delhi: Population Council.

Jejeebhoy, S. J., Kalyanwala, S., Zavier, A. F., Kumar, R., & Jha, N. (2010). Experience seeking abortion among unmarried young women in Bihar and Jharkhand, India: Delays and disadvantages. *Reproductive Health Matters, 18*(35), 163–174.

Jejeebhoy, S. J., Santhya, K. G., & Sabarwal, S. (2013). *Gender-based violence: A qualitative exploration of norms, experiences and positive deviance*. New Delhi: Population Council.

Jejeebhoy, S. J., Santhya, K. G., Singh, S. K., Rampal, S., & Saxena, K. (2014a). *Provision of adolescent reproductive and sexual health services in India: Provider perspectives*. New Delhi: Population Council.

Jejeebhoy, S. J., Santhya, K. G., & Zavier, A. J. (2014b). Demand for contraception to delay first pregnancy among young married women in India. *Studies in Family Planning, 45*(2), 183–201.

Joseph, N., Shetty, B., Hasreen, F., Ishwarya, R., Baniya, M., Sachdeva, S., & Agarwal, S. (2015). Awareness and attitudes toward emergency contraceptives among college students in South India. *The Journal of Obstetrics and Gynecology of India, 66*(1), 363–369.

Kakani, A., & Jaiswal, A. (2012). Awareness level of family planning methods in adolescent girls of different socio-economic groups in rural sectors, in Central India. *International Journal of Reproduction, Contraception, Obstetrics and Gynecology, 1*(1), 3–6.

Kalyanwala, S., Zavier, A. J. F., & Jejeebhoy, S. (2010). *Public health facilities and women's access to abortion: A situational analysis in Maharashtra and Rajasthan*. New Delhi: Population Council.

Kamaljit, K., Arora, B., Singh, K. G., & Neki, N. S. (2012). Social beliefs and practices associated with menstrual hygiene among adolescent girls of Amritsar, Punjab, India. *Journal of International Sciences Academy, 25*(2), 69–70.

Kamath, R., Ghosh, D., Lena, A., & Chandrasekaran, V. (2013). A study on knowledge and practices regarding menstrual hygiene among rural and urban adolescent girls in Udupi taluk, Manipal, India. *Global Journal of Medicine and Public Health, 2*(4), 1–9.

Kamini, S., & Avvaru, K. V. (2014). Teenage pregnancy: Maternal and fetal outcomes. *IOSR Journal of Dental and Medical Sciences (IOSR-JDMS), 1*(13), 41–44.

Kansal, S., Singh, S., & Kumar, A. (2017). Awareness of legal and social issues related to reproductive health among adolescent girls in rural Varanasi. *Indian Journal of Public Health, 61*(1), 26–32.

Kesterton, A. J., Cleland, J., Sloggett, A., & Ronsmans, C. (2010). Institutional delivery in rural India: The relative importance of accessibility and economic status. *BMC Pregnancy and Childbirth, 10*(1), 30.

Kotian, S. M., Chaudhary, V. K., Mutya, V. S., Sekhon, A. S., Sriraman, S., & Prasad, P. (2017). Assessment of knowledge, practice and perception of menstruation among adult women in the reproductive age group, in Mangalore, India. *International Journal of Reproduction, Contraception, Obstetrics and Gynecology, 6*(10), 4595–4601.

Kumar, A., Singh, T., Basu, S., Pandey, S., & Bhargava, V. (2007). Outcome of teenage pregnancy. *The Indian Journal of Pediatrics, 74*(10), 927–931.

Kusuma, M. L., & Ahmed, M. (2016). Awareness, perception and practices of government pre-university adolescent girls regarding menstruation in Mysore city, India. *International Journal Of Community Medicine And Public Health, 3*(6), 1593–1599.

Lala, M. M. (2014). Orphans of the HIV epidemic: The challenges from toddlerhood to adolescence and beyond. *Journal of the International AIDS Society, 17*(4Suppl 3), 19483.

Law Commission of India. (2008). *Proposal to amend the prohibition of child marriage act, 2006 and other allied laws (Report no. 205)*. New Delhi: Law Commission of India, Government of India.

Lim, S. S., Dandona, L., Hoisington, J. A., James, S. L., Hogan, M. C., & Gakidou, E. (2010). India's Janani Suraksha Yojana, a conditional cash transfer programme to increase births in health facilities: An impact evaluation. *The Lancet, 375*(9730), 2009–2023.

Mahajan, P., & Sharma, N. (2005a). Parents attitude towards imparting sex education to their adolescent girls. *Anthropologist, 7*(3), 197–199.

Mahajan, P., & Sharma, N. (2005b). Awareness level of adolescent girls regarding HIV/AIDS (a comparative study of rural and urban areas of Jammu). *Journal of Human Ecology, 17*(4), 313–314.

Mahanta, T. G., Boruah, M., Singh, V. K., Gogoi, P., Rane, T., & Mahanta, B. N. (2016). Effect of social and behavior change communication by using infotainment in community perception of adolescent girls for reproductive and sexual health care in high priority districts of Assam. *Clinical Epidemiology and Global Health, 4*(3), 133–139.

Mason, L., Sivakami, M., Thakur, H., Kakade, N., Beauman, A., Alexander, K. T., van Eijke, A. M., Laserson, K. F., Thakkar, M. B., & Phillips-Howard, P. A. (2017). 'We do not know': A qualitative study exploring boys perceptions of menstruation in India. *Reproductive Health, 14*(1), 174. https://doi.org/10.1186/s12978-017-0435-x.

Mathur, S., Greene, M., & Malhotra, A. (2003). *Too young to wed. The lives, rights, and health of young married girls*. Retrieved from ICRW website http://www.icrw.org/sites/default/files/publications/Too-Young-to-Wed-the-Lives-Rights-and-Health-of-Young-Married-Girls.pdf. Accessed on 26 Sept 2016.

McManus, A., & Dhar, L. (2008). Study of knowledge, perception and attitude of adolescent girls towards STIs/HIV, safer sex and sex education: (a cross sectional survey of urban adolescent school girls in South Delhi, India). *BMC Women's Health, 8*(1), 12.

Medhi, R., Das, B., Das, A., Ahmed, M., Bawri, S., & Rai, S. (2016). Adverse obstetrical and perinatal outcome in adolescent mothers associated with first birth: A hospital-based case-control study in a tertiary care hospital in North-East India. *Adolescent Health, Medicine and Therapeutics, 7*, 37–42.

Meier, E. (2003). The growth of AIDS orphans and policy solutions. *Paediatric Nursing, 29*(1), 75.

Ministry of Health and Family Welfare (MOHFW). (2000). *National population policy 2000*. New Delhi: MOHFW, Government of India.

Ministry of Health and Family Welfare (MOHFW). (2002a). *National health policy*. New Delhi: MOHFW, Government of India.

Ministry of Health and Family Welfare (MOHFW). (2002b). *The medical termination of pregnancy amendment act of 2002. No. 64 of 2002 gazette of India*. New Delhi: MOHFW, Government of India.

Ministry of Health and Family Welfare (MOHFW). (2006). *Implementation guide on RCH II: Adolescent reproductive and sexual health strategy for state and district programme managers*. New Delhi: MOHFW, Government of India.

Ministry of Health and Family Welfare (MOHFW). (2008). *School health programme*. New Delhi: MOHFW, Government of India.

Ministry of Health and Family Welfare (MOHFW). (2009). *Reproductive and sexual health of young people in India*. New Delhi: MOHFW, Government of India.

Ministry of Health and Family Welfare (MOHFW). (2014a). *Guidelines for implementation of RKSK*. New Delhi: MOHFW, Government of India.

Ministry of Health and Family Welfare (MOHFW). (2014b). *Strategy handbook, RKSK*. New Delhi: MOHFW, Government of India.

Ministry of Health and Family Welfare (MOHFW). (2016). *Revised guidelines for menstrual hygiene scheme*. New Delhi: MOHFW, Government of India.

Ministry of Health and Family Welfare (MOHFW). (2017). *National health policy*. New Delhi: MOHFW, Government of India.

Ministry of Human Resource Development (MOHRD). (2005). *Adolescence education program*. Retrieved from MOHRD website http://mhrd.gov.in/adolescence_programme. Accessed on 24 Sept 2016.

Ministry of Law and Justice (MOLJ). (2007). *The prohibition of child marriage act, 2006. No. 6 of 2007 gazette of India*. New Delhi: Ministry of Law and Justice, Government of India.

Ministry of Women and Child Development (MOWCD). (2005). *National Plan of action for children 2005*. New Delhi: MOWCD, Government of India.

Ministry of Women and Child Development (MOWCD). (2006). *Protection of women from domestic violence act, 2005. 43 of 2005 gazette of India: Extraordinary*. New Delhi: MOWCD, Government of India.

Ministry of Women and Child Development (MOWCD). (2010). *Rajiv Gandhi scheme for empowerment of adolescent girls (RGSEAG) – Sabla: Implementation guidelines for state governments/UT administrations. National plan of action for children 2005*. New Delhi: MOWCD, Government of India.

Ministry of Women and Child Development (MOWCD). (2013). *Model guidelines under section 39 of the protection of children from sexual offences act, 2012*. New Delhi: MOWCD, Government of India.

Ministry of Youth Affairs and Sports (MOYAS). (2003). *National youth policy 2003*. New Delhi: MOYAS, Government of India.

Ministry of Youth Affairs and Sports (MOYAS). (2014). *National youth policy 2014*. New Delhi: MOYAS, Government of India.

Mohammad Iliyas, C. (2016). A cross sectional study on awareness about emergency contraception among medical students in Kannur, Kerala, India. *International Journal of Community Medicine and Public Health, 3*(11), 3216–3219.

Mohanty, S., Panda, M., & Tripathi, R. M. (2016). Assessment of menstrual health among school going adolescent girls of urban slums of Berhampur, Odisha, India: A cross-sectional study. *International Journal Of Community Medicine And Public Health, 3*(12), 3440–3444.

Mudey, A. B., Prasad, M. A., Nayak, S., & Chandrakar, D. (2016). Knowledge of different aspects of menstruation between adolescent girls of rural and urban area in Wardha District in Central India: A comparative study. *PARIPEX-Indian Journal of Research, 5*(6), 26–28.

Mukhopadhyay, P., Chaudhuri, R. N., & Paul, B. (2010). Hospital-based perinatal outcomes and complications in teenage pregnancy in India. *Journal of Health, Population and Nutrition, 28*(5), 494–500.

Muralidharan, A., Patil, H., & Patnaik, S. (2015). Unpacking the policy landscape for menstrual hygiene management: Implications for school wash programmes in India. *Waterlines, 34*(1), 79–91.

Nagaraj, C., & Konapur, K. S. (2016). Effect of health education on awareness and practices related to menstruation among rural adolescent school girls in Bengaluru, Karnataka. *International Journal of Preventive and Public Health Sciences, 2*(1), 18–21.

Nair, A., & Devi, S. (2015). Obstetric outcome of teenage pregnancy in comparison with pregnant women of 20–29 years: A retrospective study. *International Journal of Reproduction, Contraception, Obstetrics and Gynecology, 4*(5), 1319–1323.

Nanda, P., Gautam, A., Verma, R., Khanna, A., Khan, N., Brahme, D., Boyle, S., & Kumar, S. (2014). *Study on masculinity, intimate partner violence and son preference in India*. New Delhi: International Center for Research on Women.

Naroor, B. R., & Tribhuwan, R. D. (2017). Determinants and outcome of early marriage among adolescents: A descriptive study. *Innovational Journal of Nursing and Healthcare, 2*(4), 177–185.

Naswa, S., & Marfatia, Y. S. (2010). Adolescent HIV/AIDS: Issues and challenges. *Indian Journal of Sexually Transmitted Diseases and AIDS, 31*(1), 1.

Nath, A. (2009). HIV/AIDS and Indian youth-a review of the literature (1980–2008). *SAHARA: Journal of Social Aspects of HIV/AIDS Research Alliance, 6*(1), 2–8.

Nath, A., & Garg, S. (2008). Adolescent friendly health services in India: A need of the hour. *Indian Journal of Medical Sciences, 62*(11), 465–472.

National AIDS Control Organisation (NACO). (2002). *National AIDS prevention and control policy*. New Delhi: NACO. Ministry of Health and Family Welfare, Government of India.

National AIDS Control Organisation (NACO). (2004). *Annual report 2002–2004*. New Delhi: NACO.

National Behavioural Surveillance Survey (BSS). (2006). *Youth (15–24 years)*. New Delhi: NACO, Ministry of Health and Family Welfare, Government of India.

National Council of Educational Research and Training (NCERT). (2011). *Training and resource materials under the adolescent education programme*. New Delhi: NCERT. Retrieved from NCERT website http://www.ncert.nic.in/programmes/aep/aep.html. Accessed on 26 Sept 2016.

National Institute of Medical Statistics and National AIDS Control Organisation (NACO). (2008).

Navaneetham, K., & Dharmalingam, A. (2002). Utilization of maternal health care services in Southern India. *Social Science and Medicine, 55*(10), 1849–1869.

Nayak, S., Toppo, N. A., Tomar, S. P., Kasar, P. K., & Tiwari, R. (2016). A study on knowledge about sexually transmitted infections (STIs) and AIDS among adolescents of rural areas of Jabalpur district. *International Journal of Medical Science and Public Health, 5*(8), 1592–1595.

Office of Registrar General, India. (2011). *Special bulletin on maternal mortality in India 2007–09*. New Delhi: Office of Registrar General, India.

Pachauri, S., & Santhya, K. G. (2002). Reproductive choices for Asian adolescents: A focus on contraceptive behavior. *International Family Planning Perspectives, 28*(4), 186–195.

Pandve, H. T., Bhawalkar, J. S., & Bhuyar, P. A. (2008). AIDS orphans: An ignored issue in India. *Indian Journal of Sexually Transmitted Diseases and AIDS, 29*(1), 47.

Parasuraman, S., Kishor, S., Singh, S. K., & Vaidehi, Y. (2009). *A profile of youth in India, National Family Health Survey (NFHS-3), India, 2006–06*. Mumbai: IIPS.

Patidar, H. (2015). Pregnancy outcomes among adolescent tribal women: Insights from South-East Rajasthan, India. *Epidemiology, Biostatistics and Public Health, 12*(2), e11165.

Patil, M. S., & Angadi, M. M. (2013). Menstrual pattern among adolescent girls in rural area of Bijapur. *Al Ameen Journal of Medical Sciences, 6*(1), 17–20.

Patil, V. V., & Udgiri, R. (2016). Menstrual hygienic practices among adolescent girls of rural North Karnataka region, India. *International Journal Of Community Medicine And Public Health, 3*(7), 1872–1876.

Patra, S. (2016). Motherhood in childhood: Addressing reproductive health hazards among adolescent married women in India. *Reproductive Health, 13*(1), 52–60.

Planning Commission. (2011). *Mid-term appraisal eleventh five year plan 2007–2012*. New Delhi: Oxford University Press.

Population Council & UNICEF. (2013). *Adolescents in India: A desk review of existing evidence and behaviours, programmes and policies*. New Delhi: UNICEF.

Prasad, J. H., Abraham, S., Kurz, K. M., George, V., Lalitha, M. K., John, R., Jayapaul, M. N. R., Shetty, N., & Joseph, A. (2005). Reproductive tract infections among young married women in Tamil Nadu. *India. International Family Planning Perspectives, 31*(2), 73–82.

Prusty, R. K., & Unisa, S. (2013). Reproductive tract infections and treatment seeking behavior among married adolescent women 15–19 years in India. *International Journal of MCH and AIDS, 2*(1), 103–110.

Raghav, P. R., Bhutani, S. T., Chaudhari, S. N., & Bamane, S. S. (2013). Teenage pregnancy: A product of various social and health factors. *Indian Medical Gazette, 147*(12), 444–447.

Rajagopal, S., & Mathur, K. (2017). 'Breaking the silence around menstruation': Experiences of adolescent girls in an urban setting in India. *Gender and Development, 25*(2), 303–317.
Rajpoot, S. S., & Gupta, K. (2016). Awareness about RTI and facts of HIV/AIDS among rural college going girls in Varanasi district. *International Journal of Home Science, 2*(3), 71–73.
Ramesh, A., Bhagwan, D., Holla, R., Unnikrishnan, B., Thapar, R., Mithra, P., Kumar, N., & Kulkarni, V. (2016). Knowledge and perception towards female feticide among adolescents of coastal South India. *National Journal of Community Medicine, 7*(9), 736–740.
Ramya, S., Rupavani, K., & Bupathy, A. (2014). Effect of educational program on premenstrual syndrome in adolescent school girls. *International Journal of Reproduction, Contraception, Obstetrics and Gynecology, 3*(1), 168–171.
Rani, M., & Bonu, S. (2003). Rural Indian women's care-seeking behavior and choice of provider for gynecological symptoms. *Studies in Family Planning, 34*(3), 173–185.
Rani, S., Ghosh, S., & Sharan, M. (2007). Maternal healthcare seeking among tribal adolescent girls in Jharkhand. *Economic and Political Weekly, 42*(48), 58–61.
Rao, K. S., Ramya, K. S., Batchu, D., & Reddy, M. P. (2017). Teenage pregnancy and its obstetric outcome. *Journal of Evidence Based Medicine and Healthcare, 4*(15), 901–904.
Raut, A. V., & Pakhare, A. (2016). Youth and sexual health: A cross-sectional study from an urban slum of Mumbai. *International Journal of Medical Science and Public Health, 5*(2), 138–141.
Ray, S., & Dasgupta, A. (2012). Determinants of menstrual hygiene among adolescents girls: A multivariate analysis. *National Journal of Community Medicine, 3*(2), 294–301.
Rudra, S., Bal, H., & Singh, S. (2013). A retrospective study of teenage pregnancy in a tertiary care hospital. *International Journal of Reproduction, Contraception, Obstetrics and Gynecology, 2*(3), 383–387.
Rupakala, B. M., Shurthi, A. G., & Nagarathnamma, R. (2013). A study on teenage pregnancy and its maternal and fetal outcome. *International Journal of Science and Research (E-ISSN 2319–7064), 5*(5), 2486–2489.
Sabarwal, S., & Santhya, K. G. (2012). Treatment-seeking for symptoms of reproductive tract infections among young women in India. *International Perspectives on Sexual and Reproductive Health, 38*(2), 90–98.
Sachan, B., Idris, M. Z., Jain, S., Kumari, R., & Singh, A. (2012). Age at menarche and menstrual problems among school-going adolescent girls of a North Indian district. *Journal of Basic and Clinical Reproductive Sciences, 1*(1–2), 56–59.
Sahay, S., Nirmalkar, A., Sane, S., Verma, A., Reddy, S., & Mehendale, S. (2013). Correlates of sex initiation among school going adolescents in Pune, India. *The Indian Journal of Pediatrics, 80*(10), 814–820.
Sajitha, B. (2017). Reproductive health issues among married adolescent girls. *International Journal of Applied Research, 3*(5), 27–30.
Santhya, K. G., & Jejeebhoy, S. J. (2003). Sexual and reproductive health needs of married adolescent girls. *Economic and Political Weekly, 37*(41), 4370–4380.
Santhya, K. G., & Jejeebhoy, S. J. (2007a). *Young people's sexual and reproductive health in India: Policies, programmes and realities*. New Delhi: Population Council.
Santhya, K. G., & Jejeebhoy, S. J. (2007b). Early marriage and HIV/AIDS: Risk factors among young women in India. *Economic and Political Weekly, 42*, 1291–1297.
Santhya, K. G., & Jejeebhoy, S. J. (2012). *The sexual and reproductive health and rights of young people in India: A review of the situation*. New Delhi: Population Council.
Santhya, K. G., Haberland, N., Ram, F., Sinha, R. K., & Mohanty, S. K. (2007). Consent and coercion: Examining unwanted sex among married young women in India. *International Family Planning Perspectives, 33*(3), 124–132.
Santhya, K. G., Jejeebhoy, S. J., & Ghosh, S. (2008). *Early marriage and sexual and reproductive health risks: Experiences of young women and men in Andhra Pradesh and Madhya Pradesh, India*. New Delhi: Population Council.

Santhya, K. G., Ram, U., Acharya, R., Jejeebhoy, S. J., Ram, F., & Singh, A. (2010). Associations between early marriage and young women's marital and reproductive health outcomes: Evidence from India. *International Perspectives on Sexual and Reproductive Health, 36*(3), 132–139.

Santhya, K. G., Acharya, R., & Jejeebhoy, S. J. (2011a). Condom use before marriage and its correlates: Evidence from India. *International Perspectives on Sexual and Reproductive Health, 37*(4), 170–180.

Santhya, K. G., Jejeebhoy, S. J., Acharya, R., & Zavier, A. F. (2011b). *Effects of the Janani Suraksha Yojana on maternal and newborn care practices: Women's experiences in Rajasthan.* New Delhi: Population Council.

Sarkar, S., Shrimal, A., Das, J., & Choudhury, S. (2013). Pattern of sexually transmitted infections: A profile from a sexually transmitted infections clinic of a tertiary care hospital of Eastern India. *Annals of Medical and Health Sciences Research, 3*(2), 206–209.

Sarkar, A. P., Mandal, R., & Ghorai, S. (2016). Premenstrual syndrome among adolescent girl students in a rural school of West Bengal, India. *International Journal of Medical Science and Public Health, 5*(03), 408–411.

Secretary-General's Report to the General Assembly, A/36/215, 1981.

Sen, A. (2005). *India is home to the largest number of AIDS orphans in the world.* Retrieved from http://infochangeindia.org/index2.php?option=com_content&do_pdf=1&id=241

Sethuraman, K., Gujjarappa, L., Kapadia-Kundu, N., Naved, R., Barua, A., Khoche, P., & Parveen, S. (2007). Delaying the first pregnancy: A survey in Maharashtra, Rajasthan and Bangladesh. *Economic and Political Weekly, 42*(44), 79–89.

Shankar, P., Dudeja, P., Gadekar, T., & Mukherji, S. (2017). Reproductive health awareness among adolescent girls of a government school in an urban slum of Pune city. *Medical Journal of Dr. DY Patil University, 10*(2), 133–137.

Sharma, S., Choudhary, S., Saluja, N., Gaur, D. R., Kumari, S., Pandey, S. M., & Hisar, H. (2016). Knowledge and practices about menstrual hygiene among school adolescent girls in Agroha village of Haryana. *Journal of Evolution of Medical and Dental Sciences, 5*(9), 389–392.

Shekhar, M., Ghosh, S., & Panda, P. (2007). Exploring safe sex awareness and sexual experiences of adolescents in Patna. *Economic and Political Weekly, 42*(48), 48–55.

Shelat, P. R., Hihoriya, N. H., & Kumbar, S. (2012). Knowledge and attitude towards the use of emergency contraceptive pills among college students. *International Journal of Basic & Clinical Pharmacology, 1*(2), 77–84.

Shinde, M., Trivedi, A., Shinde, A., & Mishra, S. K. (2017). A study of awareness regarding HIV/AIDS among secondary school students. *International Journal Of Community Medicine And Public Health, 3*(6), 1461–1465.

Shrivastav, A., Jiyani, A., & Prajapati, N. (2016). Maternal outcome in teenage pregnancy (16–19 years). *International Journal of Science and Research (E-ISSN 2319–7064), 5*(5), 1013–1015.

Shukla, M. K., Khan, S., & Srivastava, A. (2016). Common menstrual complaints and use of medication, among undergraduate students of Moradabad, Uttar Pradesh, India: A cross sectional study. *International Journal Of Community Medicine And Public Health, 3*(8), 2180–2185.

Singh, P. K., Rai, R. K., Alagarajan, M., & Singh, L. (2012). Determinants of maternity care services utilization among married adolescents in rural India. *PLoS One, 7*(2), e31666.

Sinha, K. (2011). '70% can't afford sanitary napkins, reveals study', *Times of India* [online], retrieved from Times of India website http://timesofindia.indiatimes.com/india/70-cant-afford-sanitary-napkins-reveals-study/articleshow/7344998.cms. Accessed on 1 Oct 2016.

Sinha, S., & Modi, J. N. (2014). Psychosocial aspects of changes during adolescence among school going adolescent Indian girls. *International Journal of Reproduction, Contraception, Obstetrics and Gynecology, 3*(2), 409–413.

Sinha, S., Srivastava, J. P., Sachan, B., & Singh, R. B. (2017). A study of menstrual pattern and prevalence of dysmenorrhea during menstruation among school going adolescent girls in Lucknow district, Uttar Pradesh, India. *International Journal Of Community Medicine And Public Health, 3*(5), 1200–1203.

Sjöström, S., Essén, B., Sydén, F., Gemzell-Danielsson, K., & Klingberg-Allvin, M. (2014). Medical students' attitudes and perceptions on abortion: A cross-sectional survey among medical interns in Maharastra, India. *Contraception, 90*(1), 42–46.

Sowmini, C. V. (2013). Delay in termination of pregnancy among unmarried adolescents and young women attending a tertiary hospital abortion clinic in Trivandrum, Kerala, India. *Reproductive Health Matters, 21*(41), 243–250.

Spandana, N., Reddy, K. M., & Giri, A. (2016). Teenage pregnancy – An unsafe journey towards the risky destiny. *Journal of Medical Science and Clinical Research (E-ISSN 2347-176X; P-ISSN 2455–0450), 4*(2), 9458–9462.

Sudha, S., Morrison, S., & Zhu, L. (2007). Violence against women, symptom reporting, and treatment for reproductive tract infections in Kerala state, southern India. *Health Care for Women International, 28*(3), 268–284.

Sujay, R. (2009). *Premarital sexual behaviour amongst unmarried college students of Gujarat, India* (Health and Population Innovation Fellowship Programme Working Paper No. 9). New Delhi: Population Council.

Talawar, S., & Venkatesh, G. (2013). Outcome of teenage pregnancy. *IOSR Journal of Dental and Medical Sciences, 6*(6), 81–83.

Tata Institute of Social Sciences (TISS) and United Nations Population Fund (UNFPA). (2015). *Child marriage and early motherhood: Understanding from lived experiences of young people*. Mumbai: TISS.

Thakur, N. A., & Holambe, V. M. (2016). Determinants of pre-menarcheal knowledge of menstruation and sociocultural implications in college going girls: A community-based cross-sectional study from Latur, Maharashtra. *Journal of Mahatma Gandhi Institute of Medical Sciences, 21*(1), 30–34.

Thakur, H., Aronsson, A., Bansode, S., Lundborg, C. S., Dalvie, S., & Faxelid, E. (2014). Knowledge, practices, and restrictions related to menstruation among young women from low socioeconomic community in Mumbai, India. *Frontiers in Public Health, 2*, 1–7.

Thapa, P., & Sivakami, M. (2017). Lost in transition: Menstrual experiences of intellectually disabled school-going adolescents in Delhi, India. *Waterlines, 36*(4), 317–338.

Toor, K. K. (2012). A study of the attitude of teachers, parents and adolescents towards sex education. *MIER Journal of Educational Studies, Trends and Practices, 2*(2), 177–189.

Trikha, S. (2001). Abortion scenario of adolescents in a North India city--evidence from a recent study. *Indian Journal of Community Medicine, 26*(1), 48–55.

Tripathi, N., & Sekher, T. V. (2013). Youth in India ready for sex education? Emerging evidence from national surveys. *PLoS One, 8*(8), e71584.

Tripathi, M., & Sherchand, A. (2014). Outcome of teenage pregnancy. *Journal of Universal College of Medical Sciences, 2*(2), 11–14.

UNICEF. (2012). *Girls today women tomorrow. Research highlights on knowledge, attitudes, interpersonal communication and practice on menstrual hygiene*. New Delhi: UNICEF.

Upadhyay, C., Nayak, B., & Desai, G. (2018). Knowledge and attitude of menstruation hygiene, contraception and sexual transmitted disease among school girls of Lunawada, Mahisagar, Gujarat, India. *International Journal of Reproduction, Contraception, Obstetrics and Gynecology, 7*(4), 1543–1547.

Van Eijk, A. M., Sivakami, M., Thakkar, M. B., Bauman, A., Laserson, K. F., Coates, S., & Phillips-Howard, P. A. (2016). Menstrual hygiene management among adolescent girls in India: A systematic review and meta-analysis. *BMJ Open, 6*(3), e010290.

Varghese, M. M., James, S., Ravichandran, L., Sivaprakasam, E., Palaniyandi, A., & Balaji, S. (2015). Religious restrictions and cultural taboos related to menstruation in adolescent girls: A school-based cross-sectional observational study. *Indian Journal of Child Health, 2*(4), 161–164.

Velhal, G., Kambli, T. D., & Suryawanshi, S. R. (2012). What do they know about HIV/AIDS-adolescents and young adults from slums in Mumbai, India? *SAARC Journal of Tuberculosis, Lung Diseases and HIV/AIDS, 9*(1), 26–34.

Verma, R. K., & Mahendra, V. S. (2005). Construction of masculinity in India: A gender and sexual health perspective. *Journal of Family Welfare, 50*(1), 71–78.

Verma, R. K., Pulerwitz, J., Mahendra, V., Khandekar, S., Barker, G., Fulpagare, P., & Singh, S. K. (2006). Challenging and changing gender attitudes among young men in Mumbai, India. *Reproductive Health Matters, 14*(28), 135–143.

Verma, R., Pulerwitz, J., Mahendra, V. S., Khandekar, S., Singh, A. K., Das, S. S., & Barker, G. (2008). *Promoting gender equity as a strategy to reduce HIV risk and gender-based violence among young men in India*. Washington, DC: Population Council.

Verma, R., Sinha, T., & Khanna, T. (2013). *Asia child marriage initiative: Summary of research in Bangladesh, India and Nepal*. New Delhi: ICRW and Plan Asia.

Verma, U. K., Nandan, D., & Shrotriya, V. P. (2016). A comparative study of knowledge and attitude regarding HIV/AIDS among male and female adolescents of urban slums of Agra. *National Journal of Community Medicine, 7*(2), 78–81.

Yadav, S. B., Makwana, N. R., Vadera, B. N., Dhaduk, K. M., & Gandha, K. M. (2011). Awareness of HIV/AIDS among rural youth in India: A community based cross-sectional study. *The Journal of infection in developing countries, 5*(10), 711–716.

Zavier, A. J., & Jejeebhoy, S. J. (2015). Contraceptive use and intentions among unmarried and married young women undergoing abortion in Bihar and Jharkhand, India. *Asia-Pacific Population Journal, 30*(1), 51–70.

Chapter 6
Mapping Social Innovation Among Youth and Adolescents: A Situational Assessment of Livelihood Promotion and Enhancement Initiatives in India

Sunil D. Santha, Swati Banerjee, and Devisha Sasidevan

Abstract This chapter analyses the contexts and nature of social innovations in livelihoods and skill building among youth and adolescents in India. It further explores the nature and impact of social innovations, sustainability and social value creation on the life of youth and adolescents. This paper offers a fresh and interactive perspective of social innovation. The methodology included desk review of literature, mapping of 100 organisations and programmes that had a crucial component of livelihood promotion and enhancement as a key intervention. Detailed case studies of 40 programmes were also carried out. Our analysis shows that most of these selected projects in the commencement phase are innovative. However, these projects tend to fail, owing to frequent discouragement, lack of sustained funding and absence of volunteerism. This chapter advocates the need for institutional innovations and proactive multi-stakeholder partnerships in designing and implementing adolescent- and youth-oriented livelihood enhancement projects at the level of policymaking and implementation.

Keywords Social innovation · Youth and adolescents · Livelihoods · Skill building

6.1 Introduction

The primary aim of this paper is to locate and develop a systematic understanding of social innovations among youth and adolescents with respect to livelihoods and skill building in India. The paper is expected to contribute to a fresh, interactive understanding of social innovations that are involved in the provision of livelihood resources, goods and services for the poor and marginalised youth in the country. It also explores the nature of innovation, strategies for sustainability and social value

S. D. Santha (✉) · S. Banerjee · D. Sasidevan
Centre for Livelihoods and Social Innovation, School of Social Work, TISS, Mumbai, India
e-mail: sunilds@tiss.edu; sbanerjee@tiss.edu; devisha.sasidevan@tiss.edu

S. Bharat, G. Sethi (eds.), *Health and Wellbeing of India's Young People*,
https://doi.org/10.1007/978-981-13-6593-5_6

creation that diverse types of actors evolve and develop to bring about changes in the life of youth.

Youth today face serious challenges related to inequality and inclusion, quality and relevance of education as well as training and skills, thus putting them on a lower life trajectory from the outset (United Nations 2015). In addition, youth of lower economic and social status have both reduced educational attainment and access to decent jobs (United Nations 2015). The high rate of youth unemployment needs serious introspection by the policymakers not only to mitigate the frustrations faced by the new entrants into the workforce but also to minimise likely alienation and widespread behaviour of deviant youth across the country (Visaria 1998). The liberalisation and globalisation phase has provided both threats and opportunities to India's youth. There is potential in the youth to be the pioneers and drivers of modernisation and development, and at the same time, they can become helpless consumers of the market and its pitfalls in the absence of adequate livelihood and skill support systems (Fernandes 2006). The policy environment in India also continues to invest in formal education in the face of poor occupational outcomes among youth. Thus, youth unemployment remains high in the country (Sanghi and Srija 2014). The unemployment rate among educated youth is also high and is even higher among educated females (Sanghi and Srija 2014). The aspirations of educated youth in rural and urban areas also vary considerably (Brown 2015).

Macro-level policy shifts such as the structural adjustment policies have contributed to a sharp increase in rates of educated under- and unemployed youth and attendant social problems in the country (Jeffrey et al. 2005). There are a large number of discouraged young people who do not even look for work anymore or end up working in informal spaces for long hours for little pay and no security (Bartlett 2010). The crisis in educational quality and limited opportunities to obtain salaried employment have impacted the livelihood aspirations of marginalised youth seeking educational credentials, such as the Dalits (Jeffrey et al. 2005). Yet another concern in the context of a global risk society is whether youth are acquiring the necessary skills that could equip them to compete in today's globalised markets (Spring 2008; Hull et al. 2009). In addition, factors such as migration from villages to cities and towns will continue to influence decent work opportunities for youth and at the same time to exploitation and urban poverty, precarious legal status in destination sites, physical distance from family and social networks and exclusion from social protection measures (United Nations 2015). In this regard, the situation is worse for youth because of their disproportionally higher share in vulnerable sectors of employment (United Nations 2015). In India, for example, some 85% of youth work in the informal sector, compared to around 55% of adults (United Nations 2015).

In developing countries, adolescents and youth often lack appropriate information and positive role models for income-generating activities and possess only rudimentary skills to produce enough income to help them sustain their educational needs or fulfil their long-term occupational goals (Berry et al. 2013). In a sense, there is a deficit in accessing programmes that could provide information on vocational and educational choices, educational empowerment and encouragement and practical information on available services and opportunities (Berry et al.

2013). Policy measures, therefore, need to move beyond tokenism to building the agency of youth (Iris Knowledge Foundation 2013). The discourse should be on how to nurture and sustain the creativity of youth and empower them.

6.2 Social Innovation Among Youth and Adolescents

Social innovation can be defined as a novel solution to a social problem that is more effective, efficient, sustainable or more than existing solutions and for which the value created accrues primarily to society as a whole rather than private individuals (Phills et al. 2008). Social innovations are new ideas (products, services and models) that simultaneously meet social needs (more effectively than alternatives) and create new social relationships or collaborations (Murray et al. 2010). For improving livelihoods among adolescents and youth, social innovations not only attempt to develop technical and life skills but also seek to affect their social networks and improve access to savings, loans and markets (Sebastian et al. 2004). Programme components include vocational training, financial literacy, microfinance, micro-credit programmes, developing cooperative enterprises, promoting access to markets or infrastructure and developing institutions that advocate for workers' rights or provide networks and social support to workers (Sebastian et al. 2004).

The National Youth Policy 2014 emphasises on the capacity building of youth through delineating priority areas in education, employment, skill development and entrepreneurship (GoI 2014). Entrepreneurial training is considered as a crucial part of equipping marginalised youth with basic skills to help them develop sustainable livelihoods. Such skill sets along with financial independence have proved to enable rural adolescents and youth to complete their essential schooling and to pursue a career and prevent them from being susceptible to risks of vulnerable occupations (Berry et al. 2013). In this regard, developing the capacity of individual youth, of their organisations and of those with whom they partner is a concrete means of investing in the potential of youth and adolescents (United Nations 2015). Nevertheless, adolescent livelihood programmes are few; and they are either initiated by governments or by organisations as an extension of existing livelihood work with adults (Nanda et al. 2013). Thus, mapping innovation itself is a challenging task, as there are very limited programmes meant for adolescents and young people.

There are meaningful instances in literature, which demonstrate that the state can help to generate livelihood opportunities on a larger scale. The case of the dairy industry in India or the National Dairy Development Board is a classic example, which created job opportunities for millions of youth in the country, who were employed in the manufacture and sale of milk products (Kurien 2007). In today's contexts, there are a number of GoI schemes set up to cover the various needs of aspirant youth entrepreneurs aimed at delivering better access to credit, building private sector involvement in entrepreneurship creation and promotion and providing low-cost credit or short-term entrepreneurship training (GoI 2014). The government considers it essential for youth to have access to training, incubator support to develop and execute their ideas and the credit to finance their ventures (GoI 2014).

Several social actors also nurture the mandate to address the vulnerabilities of the unemployed youth and adolescents, whose needs are met neither by the state nor the private sector. These include the government, civil society actors (mainly non-governmental organisations and social enterprises) and corporate partners. This paper attempts to locate, develop a profile and conceptualise the typology of social innovations for youth. It has to be acknowledged that the vibrant history and diverse streams of non-governmental organisations in India do play a crucial role in the shaping up of diverse types of social innovations and their practice fields. Due to the very same reason, within the context of India, processes and institutions related to volunteerism, not-for-profit social response, corporate social responsibility, social entrepreneurship and self-help and their interlinkages gain significance. The other actors in social innovation are the non-governmental organisations and social enterprises. NGOs can be understood as voluntary and formally constituted non-profit organisations that are not related to either state or business sectors (deSouza 2010). In yet another sense, these are a subset of social organisations that receive funds from external sources to undertake development work for the articulated purpose of improvement and well-being of the poor and marginalised (Jakimow and Kilby 2006).

Social enterprises, on the other hand, are considered as private sector entities that aim to achieve social, environmental or ethical objectives by developing solutions in a bottom-up manner (McWade 2012). Moreover, they focus on specific issues (unlike many non-governmental organisations) and often depend on context-specific solutions (McWade 2012). Social enterprises in the livelihood space can be 'broadly classified into two categories: entities that promote livelihoods and entities that facilitate skill development. Livelihood promotion activities primarily include organizing the informal non-farm/farm activities sector and facilitating market linkages. Skill development primarily includes enhancing the employability of unemployed youth through structured training courses' (ADB 2012:18). Some definitions of social enterprises have emphasised on the process orientation, social embeddedness, effectuation and resource acquisition strategies of social enterprises with business or trading activities to assure its sustainability and social value (Chell et al. 2010; Domenico et al. 2010). Social enterprises are thus assumed to address social problems in innovative and entrepreneurial ways bringing both economic and social impacts in the field of activity and the society in which the social enterprises operate (Alvord et al. 2004). Nevertheless, it has been argued that the gap between these two schools (social and entrepreneurial) is yet to be bridged (Chell et al. 2010).

Moon (2007) has conceptualised corporate social responsibility (CSR) as a component of new systems of societal governance, which is characterised by self-regulations by the private sector towards social and environmental welfare, thereby compensating the business social footprint. However, studies have shown that there is not a single understanding of what CSR organisations tend to be. In this regard, Khan and Lund-Thomsen (2011) have observed that CSR practices are based on the assumption that socio-economic and environmental problems can be solved through the use of appropriate managerial practices and contribute to both wealth creation and social improvement.

6.3 Methodology

One of the key social innovation approaches related to social innovation in livelihood promotion has been based on the sustainable livelihood and asset-based approaches (Arun et al. 2011). Forging constructive relationship with the local self-government institutions that challenges the traditional approach of antipoverty programmes through participatory public action and improving the capacity building of social actors to support the functioning of participatory governance and transforming opportunities into improved livelihoods is an important feature of such social innovation (Arun et al. 2011; United Nations 2015). Mostly, it is observed that such components include the expansion of rural young people's capabilities in income-generating activities involving agriculture, access to natural resources and participation in community activities and other self-employment options (Agoramoorthy et al. 2012).

On the other hand, in the urban front, work-based training programmes, technical and vocational education and training programmes complemented by counselling services are offered to channel youth towards decent work (United Nations 2015; ILO 2012). Other prominent approaches across developing countries include devising new programmes and projects engaging youth in sustainable agriculture; promotion of technical and vocational education and training (TVET) opportunities for capacity building of adolescents and youths; promotion of apprenticeships in reputed firms, investing in technology-aided solutions including ICT; easing access to finance through microfinance; promotion of small- and medium-sized enterprises and business incubators; enhancing the scope of social protection schemes; and career counselling and legal aid services (United Nations 2015; ILO 2012; Sebastian et al. 2004).

Systematically delineating the various forms of social innovations is complex and difficult. Identifying proper indicators of social innovation by diverse social actors was found to be one such challenge. The methodology included a desk review of the literature, mapping of 100 organisations and programmes that had a crucial component of livelihood promotion and enhancement as a key intervention and the detailed case analysis of 40 programmes derived from the mapping exercise. A few innovative programmes could not be included for analysis due to lack of reliable data on their initiatives which is a limitation of this paper. To map the different types of livelihood-related social interventions by diverse actors, a preliminary desk review and analysis of 422 programmes/organisations in various sectors were undertaken (Table 6.1).

From the total 422 programmes and organisations that were identified, 54 initiatives were selected for in-depth exploration (Table 6.2). The criteria for selection

Table 6.1 Number of programmes/organisations reviewed as part of the preliminary desk review

Type of actors	No. of programme and organisations
Central government	18
State government	78
Non-governmental organisations (NGOs)	273
Corporate social responsibility (CSR)	31
Social enterprises (SEs)	22
Total	422

Table 6.2 No. of programmes/organisations identified for in-depth analysis

Type of actors	No. of programme and organisations
Govt. central	6
Govt. state	12
NGOs	13
CSR	12
Social enterprises	11
Total	54

were that these interventions worked directly with youth or adolescents and focused significantly on their livelihood promotion and enhancement. A key observation at the selection stage was that the social actors facilitating interventions did not understand or comprehend their interventions as truly social innovations and, secondly, each actor conceptualised innovations differently. Future research should explore deeper into the nature and process of conceptualising and operationalising social innovations across diverse actors and subsectors.

The desk review was aimed at identifying the key debates and discourses related to social innovation among youth and adolescents in the field of livelihoods and skill enhancement. It also aimed at mapping out the key stakeholders involved, the significant thematic areas and practice fields. Desktop research and follow-up phases with select organisations revealed that a specific kind of institutional bricolage and hybridity existed within and between the various social actors. In short, a virtual interlinkage of social actors and practice fields with a mix of community, non-governmental organisations and state and private sector characteristics was identified. The detailed findings of the study are described in the following sections.

6.4 Findings and Analysis

6.4.1 Mapping of Livelihood-Related Social Interventions Among Adolescent and Youth in India

This section describes the understanding gained from the processes of locating diverse social interventions related to the livelihoods of adolescents and youth in India. This section specifically looks at the presence or emergence of various social actors working towards the improvement of livelihoods among adolescents and youth in the past one decade in the country and explains how these have diversified to achieve the goals of improving life and livelihoods of youth and adolescents across different parts of the country.

Of the 18 *government sector programmes* that were reviewed, more than 10 programmes aimed at addressing issues of development, empowerment and promotion of employment, innovation and enterprises among youth and adolescent. However, most of these employment programmes did not have a direct focus on youth but on categories such as women, rural households where adolescents and youth are considered as a subset. The central government schemes operate across India. They work with different state governments to implement the programmes. The state government programmes are spread across the respective state and in its districts. Some programmes are seen to be functioning at the micro level as well. Though, from the primary understanding, the wide reach of the government is clearly visible, data is ambiguous on effectiveness of this spread and impact on the livelihoods of youth and adolescents. In addition, there is a need to look at the convergence of crucial schemes across diverse government departments impacting the livelihoods of adolescents and youth in the respective states.

All the identified *NGOs* (13 NGOs) implemented focused interventions among various marginalised groups including adolescents and youth. A key strategy of most of the NGOs was to implement government and CSR programmes that aim towards inter-actoral convergence as an implementation model. Most of the NGOs follow a clustered geographical approach to work with their target groups. There is a strong sense of territorialism felt among NGOs whereby each NGO operates within a geographical boundary and avoids working with a community or slum settlement if any other NGOs are operational in that part.

Eleven *social enterprises* (SEs) offering various specific services to adolescents or youth in the country were selected for analysis. Unlike their NGO counterparts, most of these SEs are characterised by both social value creation and profit orientation. Thus, when compared to the other three actors, the SEs have a completely different approach. Most of these enterprises invest and nurture social enterprises that help youth and other marginalised sections to come up with initiatives that not only benefit them but also their communities or related networks. These enterprises are a source of employment generation, and almost all have elements of social innovation in them. An important observation is that all these social enterprises provide opportunities to entrepreneurs to set up their enterprises and at the same time address a social problem such as unemployment, lack of access to education, etc. They have made these social challenges into opportunities that can be invested in, thereby initiating the process of change. In other words, SEs focus on social problems that can be converted into a market opportunity such as employment generation, alternate energy, financial inclusion and the like. The immediate beneficiaries are the marginalised sections of the population who are either social entrepreneurs themselves or are benefactors of these enterprises as employees. For example, social enterprise such as Jayaashree Industries in Tamil Nadu makes low-cost sanitary napkins for rural women. Their machines are sold in various SHGs across the country and in seven other countries. They have thus helped to create employment at the grass root level and have addressed an issue that affects adolescent girls, youth and women. Another aspect is that most of these SE's intervention spaces are rural areas.

Our observations indicate that most of the *CSR* initiatives have their roots in their parent company's values of philanthropy and volunteerism. The recent Companies Act 2013 also has paved the pathway for embedding suitable CSR initiatives for the adolescents and youth. CSR-based actors play an important role in addressing the needs of the youth with respect to demands in the job market. Most of the CSR interventions are project based, with a definite time-period of implementation. The entire life cycle of training, employment generation and follow-up factors keep changing with changes in the focus area of the CSR initiative. This raises concern over the sustainability of such interventions. Employees who volunteer to work on certain tasks facilitate most of these interventions among youth and adolescents and in many cases are not full-fledged projects by itself. Projects that involve the imparting of larger skill and vocational training focus on the demands of the market economy and do not necessarily aim at enhancing the aspirations and inherent skills and knowledge of adolescents and youth.

In continuation to the analysis of the key target groups that these social organisations addressed, a spatial analysis was carried out to compare the locations and spread off of the diverse social organisations corresponding to their target groups (Fig. 6.1). Most of the SEs while having their headquarters in a city space position

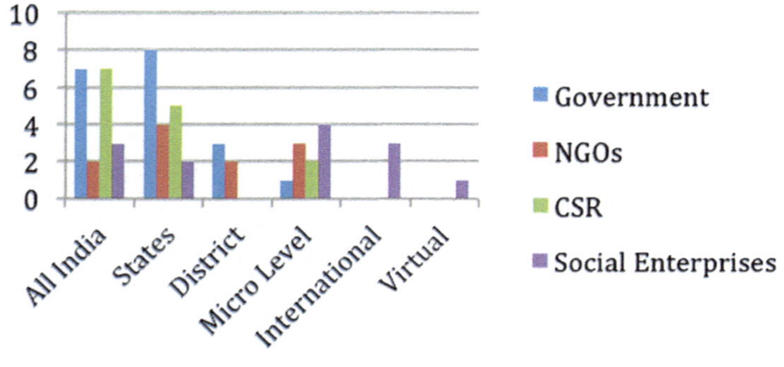

Fig. 6.1 Spread of social organisations

their sites of intervention outside the city spaces. Strategically, they seem to locate themselves in places where connectivity and visibility are evident. CSR organisations are seen to be working across India with their main offices most often located in the cities. They do work with specific locations such as rural areas and slum areas in a micro level. Social enterprises are mainly at the micro level. There are few SEs, which are seen to be present in an all India level and in the state level.

6.4.2 *Characteristics of Social Innovations*

The form in which social actors intervene is an important indicator that distinguishes them from one another and themselves (Dolhinow 2005). While some social actors offer specific and specialised services, others are involved in generic community organisation works. Most of the NGOs included for analysis are attempting to deal with practical needs rather than strategic needs. Dolhinow (2005) clarifies that practical needs include indispensable resources such as provision of potable water and other unmet needs of daily life, while the strategic needs include resources and relationships that are more political in nature with less tangible results such as better political representation. Most of them have a service provision function and were coterminous with the objectives of a welfare era. The functional focus of NGOs was thus inferred to be in the domains of vocational training, skill building, livelihood venture development, etc.

The surveyed NGOs operated in 18 livelihood subsectors. These include the provision of vocational training and skill building in the fields of tailoring, beautician, cooking and catering services. NGOs also work towards providing vocational skills on diesel mechanic/automobile repair or towards the provision of computer education, English-speaking classes and driving classes, respectively. Some NGOs work in the fields of cottage industry such as perfume making, Balwadi teacher training and training paraprofessionals in health care, carpentry, electrical work, waste recycling, retail management and microfinance, respectively.

Some key observations regarding the interventions made by NGOs are:

Social problems are attributed to structural issues linked to caste, class, gender, ethnicity, rural-urban migration, lack of access to basic needs and certain livelihood assets.

Nevertheless, the approaches to deal with these structural issues were necessarily not political in nature (in particular with those NGOs that were established in the last decade).

Most of the strategies followed by NGOs tend to homogenise vulnerable groups and offer short-term, peripheral solutions.

And often the solutions offered add up to the root causes of the problem such as lower-level skill development to feed the market.

Similar to findings shared in the literature, the surveyed SEs were having the twin objectives of social value creation along with profit motive. This has been a completely different approach, when compared to the NGOs that were surveyed. Nevertheless, it needs to be understood that the SEs are still in the nascent stage and most of these organisations were crafted with the purpose of investing and nurturing social enterprises and social ventures with a profit orientation.

Some key observations regarding the interventions made by SEs are:

Restricted to specific intervention focus such as energy, organic farming and microfinance. Emphasis on institutional building as community collectives is necessarily not a priority area.

Emphasis on bottom of the pyramid.

Nevertheless, those groups who are completely lacking access to basic livelihood resources such as landless youth may be missed out.

Social problems are seen as market-based opportunities to innovate and intervene and necessarily not addressed through the lens of socio-structural inequities.

Services and products are rendered and provision of skills and technology for the same.

For a large number of surveyed CSR initiatives, the functional focus has been generic community development, health and sanitation, finance and banking, education, environment protection, skill development, disaster relief and response, women empowerment and preserving cultural heritage. There are mainly five livelihood subsectors that the CSR initiatives focus upon. Most of the CSR initiatives aim at skill development and towards the promotion of rural entrepreneurship. A large number of CSR organisations also work in the field of agriculture and allied sectors, while some of the recent CSR initiatives also focus on microfinance and alternate energy sectors. Nevertheless, a critical observation is that most of these approaches are shallow and lead to peripheral community engagement and development. The emphasis seems to be higher towards infrastructure development projects that give better social visibility to the company such as a school building, rice mills, water tanks, solar lanterns, etc. The trend is to create visibility spaces for the company without larger social change. There is greater emphasis on skill building without institutional building or entrepreneurs. Though the focus is on the bottom of the pyramid, the approaches are a mix of obsolete community development models clubbed with modern monitoring systems.

6.4.3 Needs of Adolescents and Youth Addressed by Surveyed Social Actors

Table 6.3 reports the diverse needs of adolescents and youth offered by various actors. These are portrayed at three levels of intervention, namely, strong focus (√√√), moderate focus (√√) and less focus (√), respectively.

Table 6.3 Needs of adolescents and youth that are addressed by diverse social actors

Needs of youth and adolescents	Government	NGOs	CSR	Social enterprises
Youth and adolescent development	√	√	√√√	√
Youth leadership and personality development	√	√	√√	√√
Technical and resource development	√	√	√	√√
Skill development	√√	√√	√√√	√√
Promotion of enterprise and innovation	√	√	√	√√
Capacity building	√	√√	√√	√√
Financial inclusion	√	√	√	√√
Employment generation	√√	√√	√√	√√
Mentorship			√	√√
Poverty reduction	√	√	√√	√√

As shown in Table 6.3, the needs of youth and adolescents include development, leadership and personality development, technical and resource development, skill development, promotion of enterprise and innovation, capacity building, financial inclusion, employment generation, mentorship and poverty reduction. One needs to appreciate the fact that there is significant overlap among these needs and no strict boundaries can be drawn in defining these needs. The debate on social inclusion also gains significance in the context of the diverse needs and problems of adolescents and youth that social innovation attempts to address. Social inclusion ensures that all the individuals and groups in society have the provision of certain rights, such as employment, adequate housing, health care, education and training, etc. Analysis shows that in verbal articulation, both CSR and social enterprise organisations strive towards social inclusion of adolescents and youth. However, the data of their interventions related to social inclusion are ambiguous and lack clarity on the achieved impact. However, in NGO interventions, the whole notion of social inclusion looks at different marginalities and different group perspectives. Youth and adolescents are a part of these larger marginalities, and it necessarily does not directly place a direct emphasis on them. Nevertheless, youth as well as other marginalised sections are well captured, but their emphasis seems to be on inclusion across different age groups or similar categorisations. In CSR and SEs, this diversity is not given attention to. Yet another factor that needs to be mentioned here is that different aspects of inclusion such as issues of rurality, gender, etc. and its intersectionalities are also not looked at.

While government is seen as a key actor, the state tries to bring about social inclusion with its existing reservation policies and national policies for youth and different marginal groups. NGOs again work on issues dealing with differently abled people, Dalits, tribal population, farmers, etc., and within this, youth are also included. In the same manner, poverty reduction and women empowerment specific to youth are seen in CSR and SEs, but like in social inclusion, government and NGOs work on different marginalised groups within which youth is included. MGNREGA is an example of a government programme that has helped to provide employment opportunities to rural women which includes youth, thus leading to poverty reduction.

6.4.4 Practice Fields and Social Innovation Strategies in the Livelihood Domain

Table 6.4 briefs the practice fields followed by various actors in the livelihood domain. We have portrayed them at three levels of intervention, namely, strong focus (√√√), moderate focus (√√) and less focus (√), respectively.

Table 6.5 summarises the intervention strategies of various actors specific to livelihood promotion of adolescents and youth. The emphasis on specific intervention is placed as high emphasis (√√√), moderate emphasis (√√) and less emphasis (√). The blank cells indicate that the social actors do not intervene in that particular thematic thrust. In continuation to the discussion on type of interventions that each actor looks into, the strategies used in each of the practice fields are also analysed. The three main practice fields are youth development and empowerment, skill development and employment. Analysis shows that skill development is the current trend that is visible among all actors. Skill development is a process that helps the individuals to acquire certain skill sets that would give the individual the ability and chance to be employed and be successfully integrated into economic activities. This in turn will impact their lives and ultimately lead to their empowerment. All the actors are almost equally giving importance to this area of need. Skill development and employment are the key practice areas in the government sector. The selected NGOs for the study are seen to focus their work on skill building and employment generation with the youth. The work they carry out includes multiple practice fields that cut across education, health, nutrition and hygiene. A key facet here is that these NGOs do not look at sustaining it through livelihood promotion. There is a clear disconnect between the livelihood domains and other domains such as education, health and nutrition. Youth development and empowerment, skill development, employment and poverty eradication are the main practice fields that the CSR sector focuses on. The social enterprises also focus on youth development and empowerment, skill development, microenterprises, knowledge management and employment generation.

Employment is another main practice field across the sectors and uses strategies such as skill upgradation, training and job opportunity creation. It was also observed that micro-credit interventions specifically for youth are found to be less. Lastly,

Table 6.4 Practice fields of various actors in the livelihood domain

Practice fields	Government	NGOs	CSR	Social enterprises
Youth development and empowerment	√	√	√√√	√√
Skill development	√√√	√√	√√√	√√
Microenterprises	√	√	√	√√
Knowledge management	√	√	√	√√
Employment	√√	√√	√√	√√
Poverty eradication	√	√	√√	√
Micro-credit	√	√	√	√

Table 6.5 Intervention strategies of various actors

Actors	Strategies and design												
	Skill upgradation	Training	Job opportunity creation	Life skills education	Counselling	Career guidance	Health awareness	Technology development	Human resource development	Incubation	Financial support	Local development	Mentoring
Government	√√	√	√	√			√				√		√
NGOs	√	√	√	√				√			√		
CSR	√√	√√	√√	√√			√√				√	√	√
Social Enterprises	√√	√√	√√	√√	√	√	√	√	√√	√	√√	√	√√

poverty eradication as a practice field uses strategies such as skill development, training, job opportunity creation, life skill education, local development and mentoring. Nevertheless, largely, this field also narrows down to skill development and employment generation. Table 6.6 summarises the practice fields of various actors specific to livelihood promotion of adolescents and youth. The emphasis on specific practice field is placed as high emphasis ($\surd\surd\surd$), moderate emphasis ($\surd\surd$) and less emphasis ($\surd$).

Across all the needs except access to food and nutrition, skill development, training, job opportunity creation and life skill education are the main strategies that are being used across sectors for achieving the needs of youth and adolescents. Other strategies such as human resource development, financial support, local development, mentoring, counselling, career guidance, technology development and incubation are strategies that can be used for effective addressal of various needs. Table 6.7 summarises the strategies of various actors specific to livelihood promotion needs and problems of adolescents and youth. The emphasis on specific intervention is placed as high emphasis ($\surd\surd\surd$), moderate emphasis ($\surd\surd$) and less emphasis ($\surd$).

6.5 Nature of Social Value Created

This section briefs about the nature of social value created by different actors. Creation of skilled human resource and employment generation is seen to be the biggest social value that government has created. Social inclusion and enhancement of quality of life with education and health facilities are other social values created by the state. Social entrepreneurship, collective action and food security are other social values that are touched upon by the government. NGOs on the other hand work with various marginalised groups. However, their focus on youth and adolescents is not even, when compared to their intervention in other sectors. Nature of social value created among youth and adolescents by this sector is through generation of skilled human resources, promotion of social entrepreneurship and generation of employment. Collective youth- and adolescent-based enterprises could be one area they could focus on.

Interactions with representatives of NGOs (as part of fieldwork) revealed that these organisations strive towards the creation of diverse social values. There seems to be a moral value influencing NGOs in their interventions mostly influenced by charity and religious perspectives. Community development and empowerment of young women seems to be an important social value that is being shaped by NGOs. Observations show that there have been seldom any visible innovations in the approaches of NGOs towards ensuring sustainability. Moreover, process-led innovations seem to happen at the beginning of new community-based projects involving youth. These included strategies of participatory appraisal, awareness generation and community mobilisation.

Table 6.6 Practice fields and strategies

	Strategies and design												
Practice fields	Skill upgradation	Training	Job opportunity creation	Life skills Education	Counselling	Career guidance	Health awareness	Technology development	Human resource development	Incubation	Financial support	Local development	Mentoring
Youth development and empowerment	√√√	√√√	√√	√√√	√	√	√√	√	√√	√	√√	√√	√√
Skill development	√√√	√√√	√√√	√√√	√	√	√√	√	√√	√	√√	√√	√√
Microenterprises	√√	√√	√√	√√	√	√	√	√	√√	√	√√	√	√√
Knowledge management	√√	√√	√√	√√	√	√	√	√	√√	√	√√	√	√√
Employment	√√√	√√√	√√√	√√	√	√	√√	√	√√	√	√√	√√	√√
Poverty eradication	√√	√√	√√	√√	√	√	√	√	√	√	√	√√	√√
Micro-credit	√√	√√	√√	√√	√	√	√	√	√	√	√	√	√√

Table 6.7 Interventions with respect to needs and strategies of adolescents and youth

Needs	Strategies and design									
	Skill upgradation	Training	Job opportunity creation	Life skills education	Counselling	Career guidance	Health awareness	Technology development	Human resource development	Incubation
Youth and adolescent development	√√	√√	√√	√√	√	√	√√	√	√	√
Youth leadership and personality development	√√	√√	√√	√√	√	√	√	√	√	√
Technical and resource development	√√	√√	√√	√√	√	√	√	√	√	√
Skill development	√√	√√	√√	√√	√	√	√√	√	√	√
Promotion of enterprise and innovation	√√	√√	√√	√√	√	√	√	√	√	√
Capacity building	√√	√√	√√	√√	√	√	√√	√	√	√
Financial inclusion	√√	√√	√√	√√	√	√	√	√	√	√
Employment generation	√√	√√	√√	√√	√	√	√	√	√	√
Mentorship	√√	√√	√√	√√	√	√	√	√	√	√
Poverty reduction	√√	√√	√√	√√	√	√	√	√	√	√

Most of the SEs believe that their contributions are creating social values in terms of financial inclusion and it then spreads to other forms of human development such as access to livelihood resources and health-care services. Creating opportunities for the bottom of the pyramid to develop and discover unearthed opportunities amidst poverty is a common articulation they make. In this context, they highlight opportunities in sectors such as rural tourism and alternate energy, agricultural innovation and sustainable technology. The nature of social value created by CSR majorly is by generation of skilled human resource and creation of employment opportunities. Analysis of available reports on CSR initiatives indicates that these initiatives are generating a culture of social responsibility and good corporate citizenship.

6.6 Sustainability of Interventions

It is very important to understand how different social actors conceptualise and work towards sustainability of their interventions. For the government the highest sustainability indicator is that of its political will. This is followed by the factors shaping affordability and scale. There are other factors that are reflected such as institutional support, ownership by key stakeholders, social audit, decentralised decision-making, funding and employability.

Government support and continuous availability of funds is one main factor shaping the sustainability of NGO interventions. A significant factor that decides the functioning of NGOs is their sustainability designs. It was observed that most of the NGOs did not have any specific strategy to ensure sustainability of their interventions. It all depended on their availability of funds through project grants and donations. As a result, most of the interventions were structured as short-term programmes. Donors for NGOs involved in livelihood promotion and vocational skill building of youth were mainly found to be GoI funds. As the government rules pertaining to certificate courses mandated short-term programmes to be offered, the interventions designed by NGOs were also short term in nature. Other sources of short-term funding included international donors such as INGOs, missionary organisations, network organisations of international financial institutions such as World Bank, corporates, public and private sector banks, municipal corporations and microfinance. It was found that public fundraising events such as marathon and nature camps were some of the key strategies to secure funding to run certain projects. As mentioned earlier, these public fundraising strategies were innovative in the beginning. However, as many NGOs began to replicate the same approach, there was a sense of redundancy and duplication in these innovations. The status of NGOs today is thus in very precarious situation in terms of both innovation and sustainability. According to the representatives of these NGOs, the global financial turmoil seems to have affected the funding by international donor agencies and corporate. This shift in donor funding strategies to NGOs may also be seen with regard to the swaying of global philanthropy and aid practices to market-oriented strategies, which are today followed mostly by the SEs and the private sector.

In contrast to NGOs, almost all the SEs was found to focus only on long-term interventions, and sustainability was the key principle that they adhered to. To ensure sustainability, the SEs also customised their interventions to needs of diverse stakeholders such as investors and clients. They also design their intervention as a series of short-term ventures embedded within the long-term mode. Apart from these strategies, they design institutional spaces (say, both as not-for-profit and for-profit) that facilitate appropriate revenue generation or earned-income opportunities through their social ventures. Apart from these, they also explore traditional modes of fundraising through donations and grants. Donations for SEs were mostly through their own funding sources (which is often kept confidential), venture capitalists (individuals and companies), equity funds, partnering with like-minded organisations and co-partnerships. Thus, some of the key strategies of SEs to ensure sustainability were (1) embedding earned-income opportunities and revenue generation models within the programme design, (2) diversifying organisational forms into hybrids and (3) securing new arenas of market-based fundraising mechanisms through investments from venture capitalists and seed funders.

For CSR, ownership by key stakeholders and acquired skill sets and employability of youth trained are the main sustainability indicators. In terms of financial sustainability, CSRs have some advantages when compared to NGOs and SEs. Firstly, a committed allocation of monetary resources from the parent corporate is ensured through both the company policy and the prescribed Companies Act. Profit of the parent company is the source of donation for the projects and programmes that are run by the CSRs. In addition, the foundations and trusts nurtured by the corporates can explore other sources of funding and revenue generation as well. Secondly, the CSRs mostly rely on the volunteerism of the employees in the parent company. These volunteers are also awarded with tokens of appreciation. Nevertheless, our understanding is that sustainability of social value created has not been part of strategic management decisions. Some initiatives that were started by the CSRs have been discontinued due to recession or market instability. There have also been instances where the sustainability of any initiative whether it of a microenterprise or self-help group started by the CSR project is highly dependent on the mentoring and funding of the CSR body. This in turn has found to limit the sustaining capabilities of the very enterprises formed by the CSR.

6.7 The Way Forward

Our analysis of social innovation programmes among youth shows that most of these projects in the commencement phase are innovative; however, owing to frequent discouragement, lack of sustained funding and volunteerism, these projects are threatened to fail. One of the key gaps of such interventions is that most of these are not designed based on the needs and interests of the youth, instead are externally designed (Bartlett 2010). One of the pitfalls of the government sector is that though there is an active participation of various departments, there is no convergence between these departments. Many of the government initiatives will be more effective and efficient if there is coordination between various departments.

Questions are also raised about the employable skills rendered by existing programmes, which are a result of supply driven and not demand driven and lack of interface among different stakeholders, namely, policymakers, industry, trainers and educational institutions (Sanghi and Srija 2014). And necessarily these skill development and livelihood promotion programmes do not guarantee the empowerment of the youth (Prakash 2013). Other factors that are found to affect innovative livelihood programmes for adolescents in particular are lack of community buy-in; lack of safe spaces for engagement; gender insensitivity; inability to carve out differential programmes that target specific needs for specific groups; insensitivity to the aspiration of girl's aspirations and their practical needs; and the need to expand the scope of livelihoods beyond skill-building activities (Nanda et al. 2013).

Drawing insights from the desktop review and analysis, it is envisaged that the CoEAY could play a lead role in the following aspects:

Strengthening conceptual and theoretical foundations of adolescent- and youth-specific social innovations.

Establishing multi-stakeholder partnerships in designing and implementing adolescent- and youth-oriented livelihood promotion and enhancement projects.

Undertaking evidence-based, empirical research on the livelihood struggles and success stories of adolescents and youth, across spatial-segmental-sectoral dimensions.

Emerging as a think-tank, design and incubation hub in the domain of adolescent- and youth-specific livelihoods.

Facilitating action research projects in developing practice-based models of livelihood promotion and enhancement for adolescents and youth. These models should further feed into policy development.

Organising certificate-based training programmes, round-tables and workshops for youth and adolescents (and on youth and adolescents) towards improving the capabilities and capacities of adolescents, youth and professionals in the field.

Engaging in the consistent publication of CoEAY working papers and case studies. Some of the themes to begin with could be climate change and youth, social entrepreneurship development, employability and work readiness of adolescents and youth, deconstructing skill development, documenting social innovation cases among youth and adolescents, development transitions, marginalisation and aspirations of youth, migration, youth and cities, etc.

References

ADB. (2012). *India social enterprise: Landscape report*. Mandaluyong: Asian Development Bank.

Agoramoorthy, G., Hsu, M. J., & Shieh, P. (2012). India's women-led vegetable cultivation improves economic and environmental sustainability. *Scottish Geographical Journal, 128*(2), 87–99.

Alvord, S. H., Brown, L. D., & Letts, C. W. (2004). Social entrepreneurship and societal transformation: An exploratory study. *The Journal of Applied Behavioral Science, 40*(3), 260–282.
Arun, S., Arun, T., & Devi, U. (2011). Transforming livelihoods and assets through participatory approaches: The Kudumbashree in Kerala, India. *International Journal of Public Administration, 34*(3), 171–179.
Bartlett, S. (2010). Editorial: Responding to urban youth's own perspectives. *Environment and Urbanisation, 22*(2), 307–316.
Berry, M. O., Kuriansky, J., Little, M. C., Vistman, B., Mosisili, M. S., Hlothoane, L., Matlanyane, M., Mokobori, T., Mosuhli, S., & Pebane, J. (2013). Entrepreneurial training for girls empowerment in Lesotho: A process evaluation of a model programme. *South Africa Journal of Psychology, 43*(4), 445–458.
Brown, T. (2015). Youth mobilities and rural–urban tensions in Darjeeling, India, South Asia. *Journal of South Asian Studies, 38*(2), 263–275.
Chell, E., Nicolopoulou, K., & Karatas-Ozkan, M. (2010). Social entrepreneurship: Innovation and cross-cultural aspects. *Entrepreneurship and Regional Development, 22*(6), 485–494.
de Souza, R. (2010). NGOs in India's elite newspapers: A framing analysis. *Asian Journal of Communication, 20*(4), 477–493.
Dolhinow, R. (2005). Caught in the middle: The state, NGOs and the limits to grassroots organising along the US-Mexico border. In N. Laurie & L. Bondi (Eds.), *Working the spaces of neoliberalism* (pp. 164–185). Malden: Blackwell Publishing.
Domenico, M. D., Haugh, H., & Tracey, P. (2010). Social bricolage: Theorising social value creation in social enterprises. *Entrepreneurship Theory and Practice, 34*(4), 681–703.
Fernandes, L. (2006). *India's new middle class: Democratic politics in an era*. Minneapolis: University of Minnesota Press.
GoI. (2014). *National Youth Policy 2014*. Ministry of Youth Affairs and Sports, Government of India. Accessed at http://yas.nic.in/sites/default/files/National-Youth-Policy-Document.pdf. Accessed 1 July 2017.
Hull, G., Zacher, J., & Hibbert, L. (2009). Youth, risk and equity in a global world. *Review of Research in Education, 33*(1), 117–159.
ILO. (2012). *The youth employment crisis: Time for action*. Report V, International Labour Conference, 101st Session. Geneva: International Labour Office.
IRIS Knowledge Foundation. (2013). *State of the urban youth, India 2012: Employment, livelihood and skills*. Mumbai: IRIS Knowledge Foundation and UN Habitat. Accessed at http://www.esocialsciences.org/general/a201341118517_19.pdf. Last accessed 1 July 2017.
Jakimow, T., & Kilby, P. (2006). Empowering women: A critique of the blueprint of self-help groups in India. *Indian Journal of Gender Studies, 13*(3), 375–400.
Jeffrey, C., Jeffrey, P., & Jeffrey, R. (2005). When schooling fails: Young men, education and low-caste politics in rural north India. *Contributions to Indian Sociology, 39*(1), 1–38.
Khan, F. R., & Lund-Thomsen, P. (2011). CSR as imperialism: Towards a phenomenological approach to CSR in the developing world. *Journal of Change Management, 11*(1), 73–90.
Kurien, V. (2007). India's milk revolution: Investing in rural producer organizations. In D. Narayan & E. Glinskaya (Eds.), *Ending poverty in South Asia: Ideas that work* (pp. 37–67). Washington, DC: The World Bank.
McWade, W. (2012). The role of social enterprises and social investors in the development struggle. *Journal of Social Entrepreneurship, 3*(1), 96–112.
Moon, J. (2007). The contribution of corporate social responsibility to sustainable development. *Sustainable Development, 15*(5), 296–306.
Murray, R., Caulier-Grice, J., & Mulgan, G. (2010). *The open book of social innovation*. London: NESTA and Young Foundation.
Nanda, P., Das, P., Singh, A., & Negi, R. (2013). *Addressing comprehensive needs of adolescent girls in India: A potential for creating livelihoods*, New Delhi: International Centre for Research on Women. Accessed at https://www.icrw.org/wp-content/uploads/2016/10/Adolescent-Girls_22ndMar13.pdf. Last accessed 1 July 2017.

Phills, J. A., Deiglmeier, K., & Miller, D. T. (2008) Rediscovering Social Innovation. *Stanford Social Innovation Review*, Fall 2008. Accessed at https://ssir.org/images/articles/2008FA_feature_phills_deiglmeier_miller.pdf. Last accessed 1 July 2017.

Prakash, P. (2013). *Towards a youth agency in policy and practice, in State of the Urban Youth in India 2012*. Mumbai: Iris Knowledge Foundation and UN-Habitat, (1–6). Accessed at http://www.esocialsciences.org/general/a201341118517_19.pdf. Last accessed 1 July 2017.

Sanghi, S., & Srija, A. (2014). *Youth unemployment in India*. Bulletin, Confederation of Indian Industry, pp. 33–38.

Sebastian, M. P., Grant, M., & Mensch, B. (2004). *Integrating adolescent livelihood activities within a reproductive health programme for urban slum dwellers in India*. New Delhi: Population Council, CARE and CORT.

Spring, J. (2008). Research on globalization and education. *Review of Educational Research, 78*(2), 330–363.

United Nations. (2015). *Switched on: Youth at the heart of sustainable development in Asia and the Pacific*. Regional Coordination Mechanism – United Nations Development Group, Asia-Pacific Thematic Working Group on Youth, Bangkok. Accessed at http://www.unescap.org/sites/default/files/Switched%20On.pdf. Last accessed 1 July 2017.

Visaria, P. (1998). *Unemployment among youth in India: Level, nature and policy implications* (Employment and Training Papers 36). Geneva: International Labour Office. Accessed at http://www.ilo.org/wcmsp5/groups/public/%2D%2D-ed_emp/documents/publication/wcms_120233.pdf. Last accessed 1 July 2017.

Chapter 7
Researching Adolescents and Youth in India: An Assessment of Data Quality and Research Capacity

Geeta Sethi and Shalini Bharat

Abstract Understanding adolescents and youth and the determinants of their health and well-being requires in-depth, inter-sectoral, contextualised empirical data. Reviews of studies on four thematic areas related to adolescents and youth revealed that such research is not readily available in the country, and there are major gaps in information related to young people. This chapter examines the need for data and issues related to quality of available data, including capacity to undertake research with adolescents and youth. A qualitative study was undertaken with academics and heads of select national and international organisations working in the broad areas of health in India, who train and employ researchers, to examine quality issues in research and understand the requirements for building research capacity of scholars and career researchers. Findings revealed a range of issues in developing and consolidating this capacity and the difficulties faced therein. The chapter elaborates on the different skills/attributes required for research, particularly with adolescents, and the structural and other challenges in building this capacity. It concludes with summarising positive approaches that have worked and makes suggestions for the way forward.

Keywords Adolescents and youth · Research · Capacity building · Training

G. Sethi (✉)
Centre of Excellence on Adolescents and Youth, Tata Institute of Social Sciences, Mumbai, Maharashtra, India
e-mail: geeta.sethi@tiss.edu

S. Bharat
Director, Tata Institute of Social Sciences, Mumbai, Maharashtra, India

S. Bharat, G. Sethi (eds.), *Health and Wellbeing of India's Young People*,
https://doi.org/10.1007/978-981-13-6593-5_7

7.1 Introduction

Adolescent- and youth-centred policies and programmes require a deep understanding of the determinants of health, productivity and well-being of young people and complex and nuanced analyses of the context in which these unfold. Such analyses must necessarily be based on an empirically sound data base that is inter-sectoral and context specific, to take into account the vast range of differences in the country. Simultaneously, a deeper exploration of the perspectives, experiences and aspirations of the diverse and heterogeneous population of adolescents and youth is also necessary. In other words, to be effective and feasible, sound forward-looking policies and programmes must be based on credible, multisectoral evidence that draws on biological, social, psychological, economic and political frameworks. As far as possible, this evidence must include adolescents and youth in its design, operationalisation and analysis. Further, to maximise impact and cost-effectiveness, well thought-out programmes must be implemented to scale in an inclusive and accountable manner, regularly monitored and revised in accordance with the findings of the assessments. However, designing such inclusive- and youth-centred policies and programmes requires robust data, qualitative as well as quantitative, that capture the changing context, sociocultural contours, rapidly evolving technology and experiences and aspirations of adolescents and youth in contemporary India. It also requires a mind-set which acknowledges the high importance of inclusiveness of young people as well as of accountability to their constituency, in research endeavours relevant to them.

Adolescents and youth undergo several transitions: biological and physical, with growth and maturation of the body; neurological, with development of the brain and an expansion in the capacity to make decisions that consider multiple factors; social, with increasing significance of peers in their lives and the development of altruism; psychological, with the development of extreme consciousness of their body image and of how they are perceived by others along with an acute sense of self-stigma; and from dependent consumers to productive workers with all the varied demands and discipline of a workplace. Different kinds of preparation and support are required to ensure these transitions are as smooth and positive as possible, especially as they are now occurring in a rapidly changing social context. For example, adolescents and young people are more likely to migrate and live in a very different world from that of their parents, they are more comfortable with the use of social media, and their contacts and influencers extend far beyond their immediate social circles and across different geographies. Hence, understanding what shapes their world and lives is both complex and multilayered.

Sound evidence on these dimensions that intertwine to shape the well-being and development as well as opportunities for adolescents and youth, along with an assessment of the social and structural determinants of well-being, are required to design appropriate nurturing and supportive programmes. Adolescents and youth also require value-based and sociocultural information and guidance to enable them to transition into healthy, happy and integrated adult members of families and communities. Understanding how this information and guidance could be made effectively accessible, acceptable and actionable to adolescents and youth along with understanding the functioning and dynamics of new communication media and credible messengers is also critical to developing the potentials of young people.

7.1.1 *The Context of the Study*

A review of the existing research on adolescents and youth in four thematic areas, viz. nutrition, sexual and reproductive health, mental health and livelihoods (see Chaps. 2, 3, 4, 5 and 6), highlighted the limitations and inadequacy of available Indian data to meet the needs of program and policy-makers as outlined above. To begin with, issues with regard to data are summarised here: Firstly, data disaggregated by age and gender is not easily available for most of the important variables. Age-based data, when reported, is often available for varying age ranges rendering data comparability across studies quite difficult. For example, adolescents and youth can best be studied as a trichotomy of 5-year age ranges: young adolescents aged 10–14 years, older adolescents aged 15–19 years and youth aged 20–24 years. Each stage is marked by differences in development as well as in the priority of different issues, for example, psychosexual identity maybe more important at 10–14 years of age and skills for an economically productive role more important at 20–24 years of age. However, there are often overlaps in age groups reported in studies, with different researchers and departments using different definitions and categorisation for "adolescents" (9–13/10–15, etc.) and "youth" (19–24/18–30, etc.). The emphasis on girls, the girl child and women, has resulted in a significant body of research on female adolescents and young women but comparatively little on boys/men. Additionally, the available data is often strictly sectoral, and defined, collected and analysed in a particular framework, and not easily available in formats that are amenable to analysis across disciplines and sectors.

The Youth Study conducted by the Population Council and International Institute of Population Sciences across six states from 2004 to 2010 provided thought-provoking data on the realities of youth aged 15–29 years. That this kind of robust up-to-date data on India's young people, disaggregated by age, geography, gender and other socio-economic and cultural variables, is not readily available may be attributable to a number of factors. A key issue, as mentioned above, is that adolescence and youth are not uniformly defined, and there is no commonly agreed understanding of these terms. This lack of conceptual clarity is at least partially because adolescence and youth as research themes are not accorded sufficient importance in the country. The result is inadequate conceptual clarity in definitions and segmentation. Further, to a large extent, adolescents and young people in India, especially younger adolescents aged 10–16 years, are not expected to have opinions, views and perspectives on major issues. Therefore, it has not been deemed necessary to consider their views in a serious manner in planning and programming. Often, parents, teachers, community leaders or other "guardians", adult stakeholders in the lives of adolescents, are seen as more reliable sources of information regarding adolescents, rather than the young people themselves. There is also a lack of appropriate methodologies and research tools to collect information from adolescents. Many adolescents may not be sufficiently articulate or possess the vocabulary to describe their thoughts, feelings and views, especially on sensitive topics. Cultural boundaries, inhibitions around discussing certain topics, especially with adult researchers, as well as the social distance between adult researchers and young respondents, make exploring the views and feeling of adolescents difficult and challenging. Lack of adequate understanding and skills in dealing with ethical issues around probing sensitive and personal topics with adolescents, including those related to mental health, sexual and reproductive health as well as experiences of violence, abuse and different kinds of ill-treatment or denial of rights, also discourages researchers from doing adolescent-centred research. For example, lack of proper skills may prohibit direct questioning of adolescents about sensitive topics unless an adult is present. And yet, having an adult from the immediate social circle present during data collection may further inhibit honest responses, especially if adults within or close to the family or school are part of the problem. Most researchers do not think it important to consult young people during the research design phase which means that issues specifically relevant to them are not formulated, researched and understood from their perspective. Exclusion of adolescents and youth results in the exclusion of key perspectives and data. Of special attention is the lack of representation of vulnerable and marginalised adolescents in research. Often studies on adolescents and youth utilise convenient sampling frames such as school or college enrolment lists, or youth club members, leaving out those who are on the street, out of the education system or other networks. Another issue relates to non-differentiated grouping of research on adolescents and young people. For instance, most often available research on younger adolescents is clubbed together with research on children, and for youth under the section on adults. Further, a considerable amount of research on adolescents is subsumed within a larger "vulnerable population", such as pregnant women/mothers or scheduled castes/tribes. In short, research on and about young people is limited by inadequacies of definitions, methodologies as well as special ethical concerns. Further, recording and storing data on adolescents and youth in sufficiently secure, confidential ways, analysing the findings without being judgemental and ensuring no harm or stigma accrues to the respondents also pose challenges. Finally, researchers need to share the outcomes of research on young people in ways that are positive, productive and not perceived as a threat by established institutions, leading to a backlash on adolescents and young people or those working with them.

Concerned with the paucity of comprehensive, usable data on adolescents and youth, and recognising that the kind of research required calls for special skills, sensitivity and rigour, we undertook a qualitative study to assess concerns of research organisations, university departments and programme implementers working on issues and themes concerning adolescents and youth, regarding data quality, availability of qualified research staff and research training needs. The primary objective was to gather insights into the requirements for building research capacity, the issues in developing and consolidating this capacity and the difficulties faced therein, particularly in the context of the domain of adolescents and youth. Additionally, the aim was to summarise some of the practical solutions being applied on the ground in the hope that this paves the way forward for those who would like to build such capacities in young researchers.

7.2 Methodology

The assessment was carried out during August–September 2016 in New Delhi and Mumbai. In-depth individual interviews were conducted in these two cities with a range of researchers with considerable expertise and experience of focused work on adolescents' and youth's health and development. Those interviewed were drawn from seven purposively selected national (2) and international, multilateral and bilateral (5) agencies in the development sector and social science faculty who train and employ researchers. In addition, one focus group discussion was held with select academics and project leaders to enrich understanding and substantiate early insights. Additional in-depth individual interviews (4) were also conducted with civil society organisations and community-based organisations working with adolescents and youth, particularly the marginalised and vulnerable – drug users, LGBTQ (lesbian, gay, bisexual, trans and queer) – and those who live in slums and on pavements. The need for additional data or data gaps in research on adolescents and youth and experiences in doing research on this group were also explored.

The in-depth discussions concentrated on understanding the expectations from young researchers and attributes required to effectively conduct research with adolescents and young people, the level of competence of young researchers in doing research on themes concerning adolescents; the experience of recruiting, orienting/in-house training and retaining young researchers; and the ease of recruiting persons who are a good fit for research needs and who can ensure quality outcomes in research. In addition, views were elicited on the present environment for research on adolescents and youth and the intensity of the demand for research that will inform and guide policy and programming. While the interviews were conducted to specifically focus on research related to adolescents and youth, several other important issues emerged which are more general in nature and apply to all social science research. These are included here because they contextualise the general status of research competence in the social sector in the country, within which research on adolescents and youth is situated.

7.3 Findings

The findings of this qualitative assessment are organised around three broad themes as presented below.

7.3.1 Research Staff Recruitment and Retention

There was general consensus that researchers working on themes associated with adolescents and young people need to have a certain level of maturity and understanding of issues concerning this segment of the population. Most organisations therefore prefer to hire researchers with some experience of working with young people, as this adds tremendously to their understanding of the field situation as well as their ability to relate to various situations and persons. In terms of preference for relevant degrees for recruiting researchers to work with adolescents and young people, most participants preferred MPH degree holders from universities outside India, particularly the USA and UK, as well as medical graduates with an interest in social research. Among Indian universities, International Institute of Population Sciences (IIPS) and Tata Institute of Social Sciences (TISS), both in Mumbai, were mentioned by almost all as the preferred source universities. Some also mentioned Jawaharlal Nehru University (JNU), Delhi, and Centre for Development Studies (CDS), Thiruvananthapuram, and one organisation prefers to recruit its own alumni from an in-house training programme. Most respondents felt there is a limited pool of researchers in the country to draw from, and, in order to develop a cadre of high-quality researchers, there needs to be more systematic and deliberate transference of on-the-job learning to junior researchers.

Recruitment processes at nearly all organisations included a written test, in addition to holding personal interviews. The assessment of scientific writing skills of potential researchers was considered important as good writing skills were seen as essential to doing quality research. Candidates, especially those with degrees from universities in India, were generally found wanting in writing skills. Previous experience of work with young people was considered especially useful as a foundation to build on when competencies were sought to be developed through in-house trainings.

Explaining reasons for paucity of quality research staff, respondents highlighted many issues related to both demand and supply. For example, they pointed out that since most research undertaken is on a contractual basis, researchers are hired for a short period of time, generally for the duration of the project. Retaining good researchers therefore becomes a major challenge as those with strong skills are in demand from other similar organisations. Project-based short-term employment ensures that qualified and skilled staff move on as soon as the project ends. Project-based engagement of research staff has meant that research is often not a career of choice, and not many fresh graduates opt for it consciously as a first choice. When other opportunities come up, these candidates are likely to move away from research to pursue other career avenues, resulting in a need to again train a new set of candidates. The net result is that hiring researchers with adequate skill sets to work on issues concerning adolescents is challenging largely due to the project-based nature of research, as against a secured long-term engagement.

The high attrition rates are a cause for concern as research with adolescents and youth requires special skills, attitudes and perspectives, all of which take time and effort to develop. Some organisations have sought to overcome this by striving to continually generate work to retain staff and to provide staff with skills that can be more easily adapted to other similar projects, thereby continuing to get the benefits of trained staff. Others have internship programmes, to identify those who may wish to make a career in research, while a few others provide scholarships for those with an interest, along with support for publication and for ongoing training and development opportunities.

7.3.2 Skill Requirements and Gaps

There was consensus that research with adolescents, especially on sensitive areas such as gender, sexuality, substance use and mental health, requires a combination of research skills and knowledge, perspective, sensitivity and attitudes, which are generally hard to find among fresh applicants for research positions. The ability to be and be perceived as being non-judgemental and accepting the views and preferences of adolescents and youth, even when they are contrary to accepted norms or seem not suitable for their age, is essential to securing accurate information. While there was agreement that most post-graduates come with a sound understanding of research methods, there are other requirements where there is room, and indeed need, for development. One of the reasons for the perspective gap, it was pointed out, was that most post-graduate study programs in the country lack emphasis on skill building in working with special segments of populations including children, adolescents, people with HIV or other groups with special needs. This is because most Indian universities offer a generic research curriculum and lack a sufficient practice component.

Conceptualising Research One of the major gaps identified in required skill sets was the limited capacity to conceptualise a research problem and articulate relevant research questions. An in-depth understanding of adolescents and youth requires an analysis of the simultaneous and interacting influences of biological, psychosocial and larger socio-political dimensions. Framing research to include these diverse sectors, divisions and heterogeneity requires the ability to draw from and synthesise different disciplines in a meaningful way. It was pointed out that the willingness and strength to go beyond the field of specialisation and embrace other paradigms are not commonly found among research staff. Most research, then, is constrained in expanding the boundaries of knowledge as it does not go beyond the subject and thus loses the opportunity to contribute substantially to the body of knowledge on young people.

Desk Reviews Undertaking comprehensive desk reviews requires, as one respondent put it, the ability to cover both the depth and width of a topic. While it is essential to go sufficiently deep to understand the issue fully, there is also a need to go beyond one domain, to explore lateral linkages and to seek new interpretations and points of view. The expectation is that the review will open new areas and different possibilities and thus enrich the research by pushing the boundaries and making fresh connections between different pieces of information. This helps to understand the larger picture and to situate the specific issue within it. Nearly all respondents reported a lack of appetite among fresh researchers to delve deep and wide and to search for as much information as possible – pointing to the need to be more adventurous, to explore more.

Good desk reviews and comprehensive research processes require the use of multidisciplinary understanding and approaches. This is especially pertinent in comprehending the big picture, an essential for policy-related work. An ability to look beyond individual sectoral dimensions (social, economic, etc.) to the interplay of different factors is required to capture the complexity of the situation. Untangling these relationships also requires a certain flexibility and confidence to move beyond well-established frameworks to posit new connections and influences. Finally, writing up a good desk review is critical to designing a research study, but many respondents said new researchers needed grooming for this task.

Data Gathering/Interviewing An attitude of openness, enthusiasm for the subject and the willingness and patience to probe and learn were essential qualities desired in researchers who work on themes concerning adolescents and youth. Approaching these population groups without bias is a key to understanding them, and respondents agreed that this is difficult for researchers not trained for this job. The reason, according to some, was that research staff come with their own values, biases and world-view. There is an almost unconscious urge to pass these values/opinions on to younger persons and adolescents, especially when confronted with information on their lack of conformity to prevalent ways of behaving, perceiving or thinking. Researchers tend to get into a parent-child transactional relationship and have to be trained to consciously refrain from conveying approval/disapproval, positive or negative reactions to information being disclosed, and not to provide "good advice" to adolescent respondents. Building this consciousness takes time and continuous effort and requires a strong willingness to change on the part of researchers, as well as a continued consciousness of oneself and how one's own behaviour influences research outcomes.

Heads of research organisations who are constantly scouting for good research talent listed a number of attributes they look for at the time of recruitment. While data collection seems to be fairly straightforward, it is the ability to build trust with respondents, particularly groups with special needs, and with key stakeholders, that enables eliciting information otherwise difficult to access. Adolescents on the street, those using drugs or alcohol, those involved in borderline or illegal activities or activities stigmatised by society, those with different sexual orientations and those not conforming to existing sociocultural norms by, for example, forming romantic and/or sexual relationships especially with persons from different backgrounds, all require a skilled and empathetic approach of a researcher to be able to talk with confidence and honesty. Effective communication, addressing different stakeholders in ways that can build trust while still retaining objectivity, were listed by most respondents as key skills sought. Similarly, some respondents underscored the importance of understanding the information behind answers, and to record it in a language that may be different from that of the interview, as a special skill, beyond translation. Most answers are embedded in and can be understood fully only in a specific sociocultural context. Another skill set highlighted is the ability to question sufficiently in-depth to uncover the full meaning and then capture that in a language with different sets of images and idioms. This requires patience, persistence and imagination. Adolescents are likely to be wary to share openly, as they are still treading a fine line in establishing what is all right for them. Moreover, they are still undergoing transitions and therefore are not sure of their own views and stance. Thus, skills in both encouraging responses and patience and openness to uncover and explore various layers of meaning and nuance are required in research with adolescents and young people. Respondents also stressed on the ability of researchers to sort out views and ideas of significant adults who may be responding on behalf of adolescents, or are present, from those of the adolescents themselves.

Analysis is an essential step in the research process and one where there is scope to do more than is presently being done. While there was an overall feeling among respondents that this needs much improvement, some felt this requires a different level of training and maturity, and that young researchers cannot be expected to undertake serious analysis, especially identifying those elements that will influence policy-makers and programmers. However, there is a basic level of analysis that all researchers must be able to perform, and building skills in this area is required. Practical experience through field work, many felt, was a good way to build this skill, as it provides an opportunity to re-confirm the interpretation.

Presentation Related to this is the presentation of the data and analysis, as well as synthesis of different information to create a picture that will not only inform and explain the results but highlight those issues and aspects that are relevant to the context of the study. While all respondents agreed that presentation of findings and data, in appropriate visual, spoken and written formats, enhances the relevance and facilitates utilisation of the results greatly, they expressed their dissatisfaction with skill levels of junior researchers available for hiring. Skills in oral as well as visual presentation were generally poor and needed to be further strengthened.

Scientific Writing An area that all respondents agreed required serious attention, was the scientific writing skills of junior researchers. In the absence of serious writing followed by publication, sharing of the outcomes of research with the scientific and academic community remains rather limited. Nearly all respondents agreed that the rigour and attention required in scientific writing is generally not paid sufficient attention in academic institutions in the country. In addition, specialised writing of policy briefs, reports and documentation of programmes is not part of the research methods curriculum. Preparing policy briefs, for example, requires extracting relevant policy and programme inputs and presenting them in a framework that showcases different implications and courses of action, backed by evidence from other experiences. Analyses followed by reflection and syntheses are another skill that is scarce.

Experience, especially field or groundwork, makes a significant difference in moulding more rounded researchers. Those with on-the-ground experience are better able to examine adolescent issues from different perspectives, to ask questions that deepen understanding and to fine-tune questions to specific need and context. Those with greater field experience also display higher confidence and skill in dealing with the range of stakeholders and situations that present in the course of conducting research, for example, in securing the assent of guardians and stakeholders in the family and community for the research or managing any differences of opinion or ethical dilemmas.

Most respondents emphasised on the need for more training on applied research, operational research and community-based and action research within academic curricula. Those with knowledge of research funding dynamics pointed out that resources and interest are higher for research that will more directly address public health issues, identify key difficulties and indicate possible ways to resolve problem situations. There is also high interest in operations research – in finding out what works, under which circumstances programmes are effective, and identifying the factors that contribute to efficient scale up. Several programmes have been launched over the past decades with differing levels of impact. Some questions that were identified by respondents as particularly moot were: how can the outcomes of these programmes for young people be improved? How can investments in adolescents and youth ensure a brighter future at the individual level as well as sustainable development for the country? Young Indian researchers, respondents pointed out, have very little experience in such solution-oriented research, which identifies implementation barriers as well as possible options, and therefore have difficulty in adequately conceptualising it.

Finally, all our respondents mentioned the need for hard work, a willingness to apply oneself, as attributes that make for quality researchers. Along with this is a recognition of, as well as, willingness for bringing about changes in ones' own thought processes and attitudes. This enables researchers to grow and develop continuously.

7.4 The Challenges in the Field of Research

7.4.1 Capacity Development Challenges

School/College-Level Training and Examination System Some of the difficulties in training researchers to meet the gaps mentioned above were described by respondents. First, research is not seen as a preferred career option, as mentioned earlier, and therefore does not always draw students with the wide range of capacities and high levels of skills required. Further, the school education system supports and trains students to give objective answers, in short bullet points, rather than essay-type answers where explanations have to be thought through and formulated into a cogent answer. Students thus do not develop skills in writing or in framing descriptions or explanations and in expressing their own thoughts and views. This is a major disadvantage in training young researchers for research in general and research on adolescents, in particular, where the intricate interplay of various factors must be captured in a nuanced manner. The writing disadvantage is more acute in relation to research on adolescents because of the subtle nature of much of the subject matter, requiring very careful and accurate use of language, terminology, and an elaboration of findings to capture minutely graded variations and complex dynamics. Many researchers have not been prepared or trained by university curricula for such detailed, finely differentiated writing.

Language Barrier According to some respondents, while schooling in vernacular mediums helps in levelling the playing field, for a large number of Indian students, education in languages other than English limits the development of strong writing skills for research in either the language of schooling or English. Scientific writing and publication and their wider global dissemination, which take place mainly in English, seriously disadvantage researchers with limited writing skills together with lack of English language proficiency as they fall behind in publishing and presenting their work to a wider audience. The findings of studies done in local languages, which could potentially contribute significantly to the body of work on adolescents and youth, thus remain out of the public domain. Further, unfortunately, study materials and reference materials are not available in all languages, and students not used to studying in English miss out on reading widely, which would develop the broad-based multisectoral perspective that is desirable for research on adolescents and youth.

Teaching of Research Methodology While university research methodology courses continue to be biased towards quantitative research approach, teaching both quantitative and qualitative research methodology have their own challenges. Students often do not have the necessary foundation in mathematics and statistics to be able to learn and effectively apply quantitative analysis. Similarly, qualitative methods require an understanding of one's own role in the research process, a willingness and ability to examine our own values, attitudes and perspectives and how these act on the collection, analysis and interpretation of information. This necessarily requires a large investment of time and intensive inputs from faculty and students, which is not always possible in the present, pressured education system. Several of the faculty interviewed emphasised that the present system makes it difficult to develop high-quality research skills among students. Consequently, many times, students are not equipped with a sufficient foundation in research methodology to cope with high-level in-house training organised for them by employers' post recruitment and cannot derive the maximum benefit from such training. Also, the desire to work hard and spend time reading, learning and developing one's own area of interest is not strong. Most students are sharply focussed on the set curriculum and in doing well in examinations, rather than in delving deep in one's own area of interest for greater understanding and for the joy of learning. Respondents felt that not many students have a passion for research on adolescents and youth; thus developing capacity is relatively difficult, as researchers are not willing to invest sufficiently in it.

Practical Experience is invaluable in developing well-rounded researchers, and most of those interviewed said they much preferred recruiting candidates with on-the-ground work experience. The skills, ability to tease out and respond appropriately to ethical conundrums and the social acumen required to deal with clashing cultures that arise during research with adolescents and youth can be best developed through lived experience with supportive supervision. Learning programmes and situations that provide opportunities for more and more varied research as part of the training process are seen to be very useful in developing the capabilities required for research on adolescents and youth. Similarly, experience in more applied research and some attention to its ultimate utilisation, such as informing policy or evaluating the impact of programmes, could be included in training. Students would also benefit immensely from being a part of research that calls for multidisciplinary frameworks and approaches. This would give them the scope to learn how concepts can be viewed from different perspectives, as well as develop skills in collaboration that are essential to such research and its interpretation and use.

The Technology of Data Collection classification and analysis is continuously changing, with electronic devices and new software evolving rapidly. Some respondents said it is difficult for universities to upgrade technology regularly; to keep abreast of the latest developments in data collection via tablets, for example, or storage, retrieval and analysis using new software; and to train students in their use. Especially students from less well-funded institutions, as well as institutions in rural areas, are therefore at a disadvantage in developing familiarity and mastery over new technologies used in the research process. Some of the new technologies can reach across space and allow participation in research through virtual means. As adolescents and young people are comfortable using smartphones and other devices that can channel data, the new technologies and use of social media may create new opportunities for their inclusion in the research process. These need to be further developed and checked for ethical practice as well as reliability and validity. Continuous upgradation of teaching staff skills as well as in teaching new technologies is also a challenge.

Emphasis on Publication The existing university education system does not make many demands on students regarding production and publication of research in peer-reviewed reputed journals. Most respondents felt that the creation of a climate where there are higher expectations and pressures to publish could impel faculty and students to produce more work. This would also encourage them to improve their research and writing skills to an extent where publication in peer-reviewed journals is possible. Although this too is a general recommendation in relation to disseminating the findings of research, it will contribute to the availability of a larger amount of information on adolescents and young people, help draw attention to key issues and strengthen intellectual and methodological dialogue and debate on these issues.

Varied Capacities The wide variation in capacity and perspective across the country as well as in context and actual situation makes developing and teaching a standard research methodology curriculum difficult. University faculty expressed the difficulty to develop the learning and experience needed by students as the students in a class are at such widely differing levels of competence and interest, and, by and large, they have to address the needs of the less competent, as one respondent said, "the lowest common denominator". This means there is limited scope to develop very high levels of competence for those with capacity unless there is space for special methodology tutorials. There is little possibility of such special efforts in universities due to time constraints and the heavy work load on teachers, who have far too many demands on them to design and teach differentiated courses. In the absence of these graded courses, capacity is levelled off at the lowest standard, and those with higher interest may not receive adequate guidance to develop additional competencies.

7.4.2 Structural/System Challenges

Definitions Wider challenges to develop research competence for working on adolescents and youth-focused themes include those related to definitions and overall policy context in the country. There are various definitions for "adolescents" and "young people", many of which overlap. A very real difficulty in standardising definitions is that growth rates of individuals differ widely and the changes that typically mark adolescence occur at different ages in different persons. Further, there is often a disconnect between physical growth and maturation and mental/psychosocial growth and maturation within an individual. Defining adolescents is thus tricky, and while age is the most convenient measure, it may not be the most useful and accurate one. An option may be to define stages in development according to maturation milestones (e.g. menarche in girls). Perspectives such as these are not part of research training curricula, which are more generic in nature. More vibrant and open dialogue and debate on concepts and constructs related to adolescents and youth are required.

Research Frameworks and Methods In addition to definitions, research frameworks also require further development to do justice to adolescent research. As respondents pointed out, the majority of theoretical frameworks as well as tools used for collecting data are developed outside the country, in fairly different contexts, and are not always a good fit for the local situation. The research outcomes are largely not taken forward to theory building, and the disconnect continues, with a lack of frameworks for accumulating and analysing further information. More emphasis on building nationally relevant, indigenous theoretical frameworks is needed to facilitate greater application and utilisation of research findings.

Another problem is the inadequate recognition of qualitative research products as real evidence or information. This extends to an unwillingness to recognise the complex and dynamic nature of many psychosocial, cultural phenomena and to take into account the constant changes they undergo. There is a "solidification" of concepts, a tendency to stay with one way of defining them, even when there is evidence of changes in patterns of behaviour and of shifting trends in key indicators. Traditionally used definitions are often relied on and utilised, rather than accept the need for flexibility, for nuanced understanding and for finding solutions tailored to local needs.

Ethical Issues Adolescents fall in an ambiguous position between childhood and adulthood where the clarity between dependence on responsible adults and independent decision-making is blurred and is in transition. Issues related to consent, legal age of maturity and confidentiality are contentious. There is a delicate balance to be sought between including adolescents, giving them a voice and doing no harm. Who can give consent or assent for whom, under what circumstances? Is written assent always required? Are there ways to obtain answers to sensitive questions while protecting the identity of the underage respondent? These are some of the tricky ethical issues in research with adolescents which researchers face but are not trained for during their formative trainings. Our interviewees said that given the difficulties regarding consent and confidentiality, shepherding proposals through ethical review boards is challenging. It is even more challenging when the research is funded by external parties, from another country and culture and different ethical guidelines. These challenges deter potential researchers who lack the sophistication to negotiate culturally diverse frameworks for work in this area.

The Policy Environment in the country is less supportive of research, and thus funding and opportunities for research on adolescents and youth are very limited. By and large young people are seen as relatively healthy, with fewer problems. Even large national programmes allocate only a measly proportion of budget for research. Funding for research, then, largely comes from international or national research organisations, and from a few corporate entities, each of which has particular issues it would like to know more about. The findings of research, our respondents felt, especially of qualitative research, are often not taken seriously by policy-makers, who only see large-scale quantitative surveys as "real research". Educating policy-makers about the importance of qualitative data that looks at the interplay of various factors and traces their influence on the development of adolescents and youth is urgently required. Without this, the best information available will not be treated as much-needed evidence that can inform polices on adolescents and youth.

The Research Agenda set by the government is often not related to the most pressing needs and is defined through a closed, non-transparent process. We heard that the views of adolescents and youth themselves or of those who work closely with them are rarely taken into account while framing research questions. The data actually required for drafting policies and programmes for adolescents is therefore not collected. Similarly, international donors have their own priorities and agendas, not always determined by the needs in the field. This appeared to be quite frustrating for both academicians and practitioners who work with young people.

Access to Data In addition, respondents shared that it is very difficult to get access to the large data sets on adolescent populations that rest within national programmes, schemes and institutions. While a large quantity of data is routinely collected, its quality and relevance are not known. There is no systematic reviewing of programme data to assess either trends of the attributes addressed or the impact of interventions undertaken. Valuable programmatic lessons are thus not learned, and opportunities to develop guidance are lost. On the whole, those we spoke to felt there is little sharing of data, including the results of national surveys in some cases.

Missing Universities and Lack of Skill Transference There seems to be limited transference of research skills, with a small set of established researchers/research organisations getting the major assignments with high visibility and returns. University faculty and those from national research organisations felt that market research organisations and some large consulting firms are awarded a large share of commissioned research, although their approach may not be most suitable for the nature of the phenomena being studied, particularly in the case of themes associated with young people. Universities are not seen as the first choice for research as their focus is not so much on applied and operational research, and it is difficult for faculty to deliver in the tight time schedule given by those commissioning the studies. Overall, those who commission research said the quality of research produced is uneven, and it is difficult to predict and ensure, as the same organisation will produce research of widely varying quality on different occasions.

7.5 The Way Forward: Future Implications

Training Recognising that researchers require specialised training, a variety of approaches are utilised to develop the capacities deemed necessary for a specific assignment. Most organisations that regularly conduct research carry out some structured training on the subject or content of the research, as well as on the use of the specific tools of data collection. Some organisations include a component on research ethics, as well as overall methodology.

Structured training courses on specific aspects of research, such as scientific writing, were seen as particularly useful in not only developing individual capacity but also in promoting a scientific environment where excellence in research is valued, supported and practiced.

Perspective Building and Value Clarification As one of the crucial factors in quality research is attitudes and values of researchers, significant efforts are made to develop appropriate values and to strengthen understanding and internalisation of key concepts such as gender. This has been done through dedicated workshops, ongoing discussions in staff meetings and thorough demonstration or modelling by mentors and peers, in organisations we spoke to. Our interlocutors emphasised that perspective building and value clarification are ongoing processes and cannot be done in one workshop – it has to be continuous, raising consciousness about how the values are translated into day-to-day actions on a daily basis, so that it becomes a part of one's thinking and feeling. This is a major investment in young researchers but is necessary. As most organisations are unable to make the necessary investment of time and personal attention required for value clarification, this remains as an unaddressed gap among young researchers, which can impact on the quality of the research.

Mentoring of young researchers is a strategy used by some organisations, either by pairing them with a senior staff member, or with a consultant or placing them in a team where they will have the exposure to learn different skills from different team members. Those who applied this strategy reported that mentoring has potential to build varied capacities in a short time.

External Experts In some organisations, experts in various relevant areas are regularly brought in to refresh and deepen staff knowledge and skills, as well as to interact and provide inputs to the functioning of the organisation. This ongoing communication with the top minds in the field develops new perspectives as well as continuously motivates staff to do more, to learn from other experiences and to stay up to date.

Scholarships A few organisations have programmes of internship or scholarships that provide opportunities to young persons to study/work and learn and further explore their own interest and commitment to the field and to research. A budget is also provided to encourage and support researchers on scholarship to publish in reputed journals.

It is a challenge to keep young researchers motivated as they find their work repetitive. Some attempts have been made to give them greater flexibility, more opportunity to choose what they would like to work on and supportive learning teams to work with.

To Conclude our findings indicate major gaps at the conceptual as well as the skill level in the capacity to conduct research with adolescents and youth. Given the strategic importance of this segment of the population over the next several years, and that sound data is essential for planning as well as programmes, there is an urgency to build the requisite research capacity at the earliest. Based on the lacunae identified, we propose a 3-month training course to cover the following four sections:

1. **Conceptual background:** The period of adolescence and youth as marked by biological and physiological growth and change; sexual maturation and accompanying issues and challenges; neurological development and increased capacity for complex decision-making; psychosocial growth and development; changing roles and increasing social and economic agency; definitions, contextualising adolescence and youth, understanding adolescence and youth in different Indian settings; and understanding diversity, heterogeneity and the myriad transitions associated with this population.
2. **Theoretical frameworks** for framing research questions, analysis and interpretation of findings. Multisectoral and interdisciplinary dimensions of issues related to adolescents and youth and designing research that can capture the inter-twined influence of multiple factors. Inclusion of adolescents, giving them a voice, a rights-based understanding. Ensuring the most vulnerable and marginalised are represented. Introducing a trichotomy of age groups with significant attributes, for study and analysis.
3. **Value clarification and ethics** of research with adolescents: Understanding the special sensitivity of adolescents and youth. The need to challenge existing norms and assert self; sexuality, exploring sexual identity, gender and gender identity; development of self and self-hood; shame, stigma and peer-group pressures; acceptance and being non-judgemental; and ethics of research with this segment. The special considerations around age of majority and having a voice. Consent and assent. Doing no harm and articulating findings and issues in acceptable and actionable ways.
4. **Methods and skills of research:** Building rapport, in-depth interviewing, and accurate recording of responses; dealing with difficult situations during data collection, especially with parents/guardians/community leaders; comprehensive desk reviews; new technologies of data collection and data analyses; and using social media for research. Communicating the findings of research to different audiences – Scientific writing, development of policy briefs, best-practice documentation, and media hand-outs for advocacy.

The course will include a substantial practical component, where students will conduct research in the field. The course can be offered in collaboration with other universities as well as civil society organisations working with this population segment to provide greater encouragement and opportunity to research and document their work and experiences. We are confident this will propel research on adolescents and youth and provide sound evidence for the future.